THE DAVID SOLOMON CHRONICLES
BOOK II

TRAINING WIRES OF THE SOUL

A Memoir, a Message, and a Malignant Tumor

The Incredible Journey of a Writer's Race Against Time!

David Solomon
With Delynn Solomon

-Quotations from the website www.nderf.org and ww.aderf.org are printed with permission from Jeffrey Long., M/D/ and Jody Long.

Some names have been changed to protect privacy

Copyright © 2021 by David Solomon & Delynn Solomon. (DS Media Pub,, LLC). All rights reserved.

No part of this publication may be reproduced, stored in a retrieval system, or transmitted, in any form or by any means, electronic, mechanical, photocopying, recording, scanning, or otherwise, except as permitted under Section 107 or 108 of the 1976 United States Copyright Act, without the prior written permission of the publisher, or authorization through payment of the appropriate per-copy fee to the Copyright Clearance Center, Inc., 222 Rosewood Drive, Danvers, MA 01923, 978-750-8400, fax 978-646.8600, or on the Web at www.copyright.com. Requests to the publisher for permission should be addressed to the Permissions Department, Dead Saints Media, at info@deadsaints.org.

Bible Citations
Unless otherwise noted, all Scripture quotations are from the King James Version of the Holy Bible (Authorized Version). First published in 1611.

Readers should be aware that Internet Websites offered as citations and/or sources for further information may have changed or disappeared between the time this was written and when it was read. Limit of Liability/Disclaimer Warranty: While the publisher and author have used their best efforts in preparing this book, they make no representations or warranties with respect to the accuracy or completeness of the contents of this book and expressly disclaim any implied warranties of merchantability or fitness for a particular purpose. No warranty may be created or extended by sales representatives or written sales materials. The advice and strategies contained herein may not be suitable for your situation. You should consult with a professional where appropriate. Neither the publisher nor author shall be liable for any loss of profit or any other commercial damages, including but not limited to special, incidental, consequential, or other damages.

Publisher Information:
Library of Congress Control Number (Cataloging-in-Publication Data)
    Solomon, David & Delynn Solomon
    The David Solomon Chronicles: Training Wires of the Soul / David Solomon & Delynn Solomon
    Includes bibliographical references and reference notes.
    ISBN: 978-0-9972454-1-7
  1. Cancer 2. Spirituality. 3. Memoirs 4. Chemotherapy 5. Near-Death
Printed in the United States of America
First Edition

Legal Notice

The David Solomon Chronicles discuss suicide along with NDEs as part of the research. The authors DO NOT ENDORSE, ENCOURAGE OR ADVOCATE FOR SUICIDE IN ANY WAY, SHAPE OR FORM! If you are feeling depressed or suicidal, please know help is available. Though you may feel alone, YOU ARE NOT ALONE! If you are in crisis, call 911 IMMEDIATELY, or contact the Suicide Crisis Hotline in your state or country. Call 1-800-273-TALK (8255)

Dedicated to

Benjamin
&
Angela

My Beloved Children

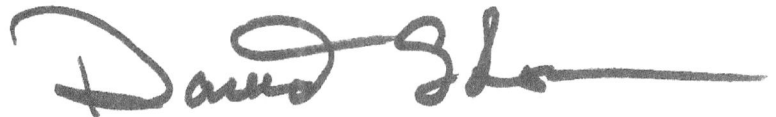

Contents

Acknowledgments

Introduction

Part I: Bonsai Sayonara

Chapter 1: Discovery: Bonsai Storm

Chapter 2: Diagnosis: Early Expiration Date

Chapter 3: Decision: 10-Day Trial

Chapter 4: Dissembling: Bonsai Mask

Chapter 5: Departing: The Garden of Cowboy Job

Chapter 6: Distance: Take Me Home Country Roads

Part II: Shaping the Bonsai – Adding the Wires

Chapter 7: Foundation Wires: California Beginnings

Chapter 8: Founders: Teacher Wires

Chapter 9: Form: Tao Wires

Chapter 10: Faculty: Earth University and a Mystery School

Chapter 11: Fold: Temple Wires

Chapter 12: Firm: Enterprise Wires

Chapter 13: Fortress: Returning Wires

Part III: The Withering Bonsai – Removing the Wires

Chapter 14: Tao: Cancer Communication

Chapter 15: Termination: The Death Wires

Chapter 16: Twister: Zen of GBM

Chapter 17: Trenches: "Live" from the Afterlife Foxhole

Chapter 18: Timekeeper: Until We Meet Again

Chapter 19: Timepiece: Dorothy's Hour Glass

Appendix: The Garden Scroll

                Obituary of David Solomon

Acknowledgments

David's gratitude to anyone and everyone he met on his journey of life are acknowledged. He loved us!

I owe my gratitude to David. He is beyond measure the most influential of any earthly teacher I have had the privilege to live with, love with, and die with. He is the best, the brightest, and the most beautiful soul who has shaped my branches in ways I never knew were possible.

My wires, gently bending along the windswept landscape of my life, growing strong roots for my soul to journey on without him by my side. The Nebari of my soul, forever grateful to have shared this lifetime with my love of my life.

I love you!
Delynn Solomon

I dedicate the publishing of this book to
Lee Gregory
David's mother for her 80th birthday,
November 15, 2020

Introduction: David Solomon

Before we begin, I must be brutally honest; finishing this book was the hardest thing I have ever done and the most beautiful thing I have ever done. Vol. I *The Zen Journey through the Christian Afterlife* and Vol II *Training Wires of the Soul* was written simultaneously and later divided and edited just as Takanohashi sensei (story in Chapter 11*) recommended from the Afterlife.

Training Wires is an entirely different book, co-authored by Delynn Solomon. We didn't know when it would be completed, but we realized I might not see its publishing. Part I, Bonsai Sayonara, is an autobiography of the beginning of my walk with brain cancer. I reveal intimate details that are the training wires of my soul. In Chapters 5 & 6, my Chronicle entries are shared—entries sifted from three leather journals I began writing when I discovered my cancer. Therein, I also recorded dreams and numerous realizations about death and dying. In Part II, Shaping the Bonsai: I expand on what has shaped my life through the many teachers in my life: my children, my family, my friends, my spiritual teachers, and my business associates. The training I received shaped my wires and prepared me for Part III. The Withering Bonsai: Removing the Wires shows the Tao and Zen of Cancer, the good, bad, and the ugly of dying and how we deal with it and finally the count down and saying goodbye. Chapter 17, *R*eporting "Live" from the Afterlife Foxhole, is magical and Chapter 18, *Until We Meet Again, is tearful.* And finally, Delynn shares some of the last days: Chapter 19, *Dorothy's Hour Glass.*

In many ways, *Training Wires* is a better book. It's emotional and dramatic, witnessing miracles, messages, and mayhem.

If you haven't read my first book, *A Zen Journey through the Christian Afterlife*, you may still be wondering, "What is a Dead Saint?" A Dead Saint is a person who has had a near-death experience and comes back to life to tell their Holy story. They have become part of a phenomenon of global proportions, precipitated by modern medical resuscitation techniques and widespread use of internet blogs to report NDEs. Where did originate the term "Dead Saint?"

In early November 2012, during my usual twenty-minute morning drive to the local 76 gas station for my favorite coffee, I was casually musing about my "near-death research" when suddenly the words *"Dead Saints" and "the Apostle Paul"* appeared, as if in a vision. In that instant, I "knew" that all my NDE research would become a book and that "Dead Saints" would be its title or a part of the title. And in that instant, I also "knew" how the book would be structured. It was inspired by Paul, the Apostle, who, 2000 years ago, wrote his Epistles directed to the "Saints." He applied the specific word to those Christians who had had an encounter with God, Christ, and divine, unconditional love. That experience transformed their lives and freed them from the fear of death.

In the end, this book is written for the bereaved mother who just lost her 25-year-old son in his sleep. It is for the father, who lost his 18-year-old daughter in a tragic car accident. This book is dedicated to the mother who lost their baby at childbirth; the son who just lost a father; the daughter who just lost her mother or the family who tragically lost a best friend. Whether you lost loved ones through tragedy, suicide, war, abortion, natural or old age, or you are dealing with your terminal illness; this book is dedicated to you.

As I leave this world, I want to share my experience with you, and it may help answer the rhetorical question, "What is it like to die?"

Part I

Bonsai Sayonara

*The truth is when my friend died,
I thought to myself, "Geeze, that's not a bad way to go. It's not
violent. Not too painful. I would have time to say goodbye to my family.
Sure, why not? That's the way I'd like to die."
My friend died of Glioblastoma Brain Cancer IV in 2007.*

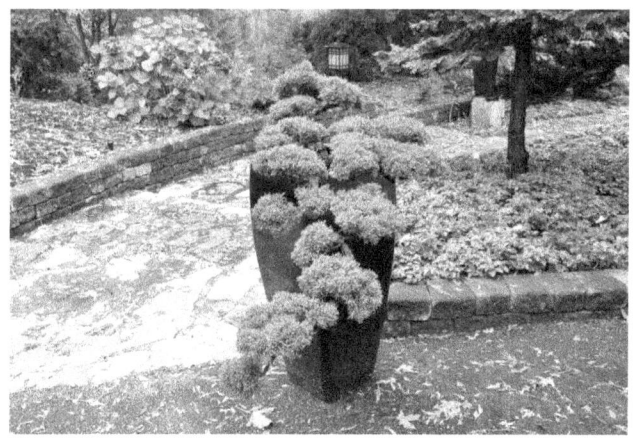

*A bonsai (tree in a pot) is expected to live the same length as the
same species found in nature. If an evergreen tree lives 100 years, a
bonsai should live at least 100 years. The life of the bonsai is dependent
upon the correct care. Caring for the bonsai includes such care as
pruning, changing the soil, and repotting as it grows. In nature, a tree
does not always live as long as expected; it can die by natural
occurrences such as a violent storm or a pestilence.*

1

The Discovery

A Bonsai Storm

Six years, four months later...
Olympia, Washington – June 10, 2013

I leaned over to pinch off tiny, green Shimpaku needles from my favorite bonsai, planted in a four-foot-high brown glazed, clay pot. Its cascading greenery created an image of a waterfall flowing over the side of a mountain. I bought the bonsai tree years earlier from Phil, who was happy that one of his favorite trees found a prominent place in Akio, my Japanese garden, and home. He mastered the art of bonsai and Japanese landscaping, including Zen rock and gravel gardens. He ran *Tsuki Nursery*, a few miles away, and we saw each other often.

I stood back to check my work. Looking underneath the tree to see if I needed to cut more, I nearly lost my balance. I felt nauseous and ran inside the house into the bathroom and vomited. My first thought was, "Geeze, did I get food poisoning from the pizza I ate for lunch?" My legs felt strangely disconnected from my body, like Pinocchio's wooden legs.

I mentioned the weird symptoms to my wife, Delynn, and she said, "Oh, that's exactly what I feel when I get vertigo." Perhaps, that's all it was. I slept on it. It was probably no big deal. Upon waking, my equilibrium imbalance had worsened. I had practiced and taught T'ai Chi for years, a martial art whose central theme was "balance," and mine was dreadfully off.

Maybe it was an inner ear infection, and all I needed was an antibiotic. The following day I drove up to the Veterans clinic in Tacoma, Washington, for an out-patient checkup. The doctor's ear probe found massive wax buildup in my ears, but no infection. He was not giving out antibiotics today, nor did he offer to remove the wax, so I drove back home with no cure. My ears were ringing, and when I walked, I felt drunk. I got out a large bottle of hydrogen peroxide, heated it, took a bulb plunger, and spent an hour cleaning out the wax in my ears. After an hour, my ears were clean, but that weird, woozy feeling didn't go away.

It worried me. I wondered if the "bad pizza" I had eaten the day before had become virally systemic, and I had contracted something dire.

The day at the medical center blurred into the early evening. After dinner, with a glass of red wine in hand, Delynn and I took a stroll through the gardens surrounding our home. Sunbeams poked through the spruce trees. Birds chirped in the cool of the evening. The sound of gravel crunching underfoot required no words to be spoken. It was an entirely peaceful night. I didn't want to ruin the evening, so I kept my thoughts to myself, hoping my symptoms were nothing to worry about.

June 13th, 2013

I did a Google search on the Internet to see if it could shed some light on my symptoms. I looked up, "Equilibrium imbalance, leg weakness, leg heaviness." Google came back with "serious symptoms. Possible stroke. Seek medical advice."

Delynn was sitting across the dining table as I pulled the Google responses back.

She advised, "Honey, I think you need to call somebody about this."

"I know. It is so odd. Maybe I've had a mini-stroke or something. I don't know. Perhaps, I should call Dr. Angelica Perry in Virginia Beach."

Delynn agreed.

Angelica was a young doctor who lived on the East Coast. I had known her since she was three years old. Now, an impressive MD, I called and answered on the second ring. She listened intently, asking all the typical questions; I didn't seem to have any of them. However, I did have strange feelings in my legs and an equilibrium imbalance. In the end, she agreed that I needed to see a doctor but that I should insist on getting an MRI.

I thanked Angelica and told Delynn that we should drive up to the Veterans Medical Center in Seattle to have the doctors look at me. It would work out perfectly because my son, Benjamin, who was 18, was preparing to fly to Tennessee for a big sales job for a cable company at midnight. After the hospital visit, it was only a short ride from there to pick him up and give him a ride to Sea-Tac Airport.

We checked into the VA emergency room at 1:30 that afternoon. I went through the usual litany of questions you get in the ER. I told them I thought I had an inner ear infection or had perhaps, at worst, a minor stroke. Anyone who has been in an Emergency Room knows it can be an all-day affair once you start the process. The doctors prodded me for several hours, checking the balance of my right leg, then my left leg, my right arm, my left. Point to your nose with your finger with eyes closed. I passed all the tests that would indicate a stroke. The most puzzling symptom was my drunken walk. I couldn't walk straight with my eyes closed, which with my Tai Chi balance, I could do any day of the week.

My head felt like a drunken man, and my legs felt disconnected from my body. I knew something was very wrong. The doctors said they were not finding anything, but they believed me. I couldn't touch my right shin to my left shin. I just poked my right heal at thin air, missing the right leg altogether. "What the hell is going on?"

At 4:30 p.m., after two resident doctors and two MD's tested, poked, shined lights in my eyes, asked what I had eaten, my medical history, and on and on… multiple times, they were finally convinced that they should order a CT-Scan of my brain. I stripped down to my underwear, and they rolled me down to the x-ray room. Inserting my skull into the giant "donut" only took a few minutes and a few micro-rads of radiation. In no time, they wheeled the gurney back to my assigned ER examination room.

Now, all we had to do was wait.

Three hours later, Dr. Ma, the M.D. on call, entered the room with a curious look of concern on her face, closing the heavy blue curtain for privacy. Something was up. The doctor rolled the short, black leather bar stool next to me, sat down, and took my hand. Delynn was lying on the exam table behind and next to me. Time seemed suspended for a moment, like a broken glass, its shimmering shards frozen in midair as you see on those car insurance commercials. She looked me directly in the eye and spoke with no hesitation, "Mr. Solomon, we found a "mass" in your brain."

Dr. Ma believed the brain tumor was possibly a Metastasis—a term that means there was likely another cancer tumor somewhere else in my body that had metastasized and spread to my brain. They wanted to keep me overnight for more tests the following day.

My response was curiously unemotional. "Well, at least I am not imagining things."

We both were stunned. Intuitively, I knew, without a doubt, the mass in my head was going to kill me. I felt calm, but inside I was a mess. My blood pressure, which usually is 115/70, was up to 146/92. It wasn't just a mass. It was worse than that. I knew it.

No matter how unafraid you are of death, when a doctor tells you that you have a potentially life-threatening disease, the news is still catastrophic. I was numb. It was just too unreal. My thoughts drifted to my son and daughter.

Suddenly I was sad. Intensely sad. I was sad for my son. I was sad for my children, who were so close to me that I might not, with these physical eyes, see their children, much less the chance to see Angela graduate or Ben go to college. I was sad for my wife, our beautiful relationship that seemed never to end. Now it appeared it was going to end.

Was there hope? The doctors had their cancer suspicions, but there was no confirmation yet. Perhaps, it was a non-cancerous brain tumor, even a rare virus, which only needed surgery to remove? With all of the drama, both Delynn and I had forgotten we were supposed to pick up Benjamin to take him to the airport. It wasn't too late. How do I tell my son I have a brain tumor the same evening he was supposed to fly to Tennessee for his first primary job to raise money for his college career?

We got Ben on the phone; I told him the seriousness of my condition and the brain tumor. I could hear the nerves in his voice, but with no hesitation, Ben agreed that he should stay home and not make the trip until we found out more information about my condition.

I hung up and cried.

A hospital room was assigned to me for the overnight stay, primarily so the doctors could do an MRI in the morning of my organs and bones to find the other cancer tumor. As you can imagine, even with my wife lying next to me on the single hospital bed, it was a sleepless night.

On Friday morning, June 14th, the thirty-minute MRI of my organ tissues the next morning came and went uneventfully. The doctors found no additional tumors. By the end of the day, the doctors were "officially" calling my brain mass a "Brain Metastasis" but were perplexed that they had not found another tumor or any type of possible cancer elsewhere in the body. They ran one more x-ray of my entire skeleton, looking for tumor cancers in the bone, but did not find anything.

The doctors concluded that I was not in any immediate danger, so with Father's Day coming up on Sunday, they sent me home with a bunch of steroids to reduce brain swelling around the "mass," and was determined I needed to see a specialist.

As you may know, scheduling for a specialist outside the VA is difficult and can typically take weeks, just for an initial consultation. Delynn began calling the VA, determined to get an appointment sooner, and with the help of the great staff (our angels) at the VA, we were immediately scheduled. We met with two specialists, and it was determined we needed to have a biopsy done. While looking at my brain scans' images, we discussed with them about Delynn's mother, who died of Glioblastoma Multiforme IV twenty years earlier. Did they suspect it could be the same thing? They didn't want to speculate but didn't think it was GBM. They scheduled me for a brain biopsy on July 1st at Swedish Hospital in Seattle.

We were restless, wondering what was ahead of us. Immediately Delynn felt the need to get things in order, cleaning, preparing for a garage sale to rid ourselves of too many possessions, anything to get her mind off of the crisis at hand. I needed to pay off a large 2010 IRS tax bill from my former company's sale in 2010. I delayed paying the tax bill due to various reasons, but suffice to say; it was the wrong financial decisions. I had invested far too much in my Japanese gardens and the remodeling of my home. I had also invested in a few different companies that yielded no return or turned out to be Ponzi schemes. The rest of my investments were in gold, and when the gold stock market crashed, my money was nearly gone. Financially, things couldn't look worse.

I was hanging on by a thread, excited just days earlier, having received a letter from a hedge fund company, ready to invest nearly a million dollars in a business plan my partners and I had presented. I had hoped to turn things around, yet, now, I was awaiting a biopsy. My life was now on hold.

An evening at the Mayflower Hotel, Seattle, WA

June 30, 2013

The evening before the surgery, Delynn and I booked a room at the Mayflower Hotel in Seattle. That evening after a lovely seafood dinner at the Palace Kitchen a few blocks away, we retired to our room. Propping several pillows against the headboard of the king-sized bed, I flopped my laptop computer on my belly and stared into the white brightness of the screen and stared at the title of *"The Dead Saints Chronicles."*

Delynn lay propped up next to me, surfing Facebook as she always does before bed. She heard me sigh again. It's a real subconscious thing I do that I often don't notice myself. She turned to me and smiled and said in her cute Tennessee accent, "How are you doing, baby?"

I checked my Samsung for the time. It was eleven p.m.

"Dang. Only an hour left until midnight. I really need to finish this final word document."

I'm the optimistic one. My glass is always half full. I could type nearly 90 wpm, so as you can imagine, my fingers fly over the keyboard, which is sometimes an extraordinary experience if you really think about it. It's a bit like playing the piano. If you think about your fingers typing too much, you begin to move from right brain, intuitive thinking, to a much slower left-brain, rational approach. When you do, you either slow down or make mistakes. It's a "flow" kind of thing. Just go with it, and it works better.

I was flowing.

My fingers continued to flit over my Toshiba keyboard with determination. I was somehow going to finish the book despite the drama and threat to my own life. Apparently, the odds were not forever in my favor.

How quickly life can change!

It was late, and I was tired. I stopped typing for a moment and focused my attention on two antique teak and green cloth high back chairs sitting facing the bed from the other side of the room. For a moment, *in my imagination*, it felt like both chairs were not just space at all, but instead sat two great spiritual beings staring at me in thoughtful repose, wondering if I might have enough spiritual vision to see them at all!

On one chair sat Paul Solomon, my deceased adopted father, and teacher, wearing his favorite Egyptian Galabia night robe, a Joseph coat of many colors. If you could see him when he was alive, he had the disposition and looked like those ancient prophets. His six-foot, big belly Santa Claus frame supported a strong, acne pockmarked face, chiseled like stone, bushy black and white beard, perfectly straight hair, and deep brown eyes spaced slightly wide apart. He just looked like some prophet out of the Bible. Yep, I imagined the old man sitting comfortably in the chair across the room smoking vanilla-laced Tobacco in an exotic Meerschaum Pipe like Sherlock Holmes. Paul used to like to smoke and think. Pipe and Paul were two peas in a pod. I've got to believe he was there watching, waiting, observing. Too much was at stake here.

On the other chair, I could only imagine sat my old Italian astronomer friend, Galileo Galilee. I loved that guy! When I was 13, I would hang painted Styrofoam planets from my bedroom ceiling, memorize every astronomical statistic, speed of rotation, revolution periodicity, number of moons, and postulate theories about the creation of the universe. I even started making my own 8" inch reflector telescopes out of a thick, oversized cardboard carpet tube. I spent months grinding my telescope mirror's parabolic curve by hand with carbon grains on a 55-gallon drum barrel. A science project I never finished. Packaged up in an old box, my mother saved for me for completion, someday, in the corner of my garage, spider webs, and all.

Galileo's imaginary ghost wasn't here to visit me on any astronomical mission, but more for theosophical and scientific support. In his day, Galileo understood that he was uncovering the truths of the world that God created. He was not at odds with his religious faith. He had immense gratitude towards God and his discoveries. Galileo believed God gave us a reason, senses, and intellect and expected us to use them as tools to interpret Scripture. He thought every truth is in agreement with all other facts and that the validity of the Bible cannot be contrary to the solid reasons and experiences of human knowledge.

Galileo was also fascinated with the Afterlife. 425 years ago, before a board of captivated professors at the Academy of Florence Italy in 1489, he answered the question no one had dared to answer in one hundred years after Dante's death; the diagram, measurement, breadth, and width of Dante's Inferno of Heaven and Hell.

During his life, Galileo equally doubted that the mass of people would be easily convinced regardless of the power of his evidence. To Galileo, the difference was significant between knowing the Truth, oneself, and convincing others:

Oh, how many consequences have I deduced, my dear Benedetto, from these observations of mine! Galileo writes again, on December 30th, 1611, "What of it? Your Reverence made me laugh by saying that even the obstinate would be convinced by these observations. You must know that to convince the reasonable and open-minded man of the Truth; these demonstrations would be enough. But to convince the obstinate who come only for vain applause of the stupid herd?" The testimony of the stars themselves would not suffice, even if the stars came to Earth and spoke for themselves."[1]

"I'm going to need you too, my friend," I whispered to myself. In general, the Church may reject the testimonies offered by most, if not all, of the Dead Saints. The implications, especially to modern Christianity, may be seen as a threat. Face-to-face visits in the afterlife with Jesus Christ, especially by ordinary people; old, young, religious, God Believers, atheists, Christians, who bring back words of great wisdom, who have no dogmatic agenda, just speak the truth. What will the preachers and priests say? The accusations, I am sure, will be tough to swallow.

My fingers lay motionless on the keyboard. I could see the battle coming. An unorthodox Christian minister with a Jewish name, trained and mentored by an itinerant Southern Baptist preacher, a Bonsai Master, and a Buddhist Priestess. What does it take for the world to

---

[1] James Reston, Jr., *Galileo, a Life.* Author. p. 133

listen to a man? A Harvard professor with Ph.D. with many letters behind your name? A pastor with a mega-church following of five thousand parishioners? Or maybe an average man who has had an experience of finding God through Jesus Christ and nature, not only in his heart and in his own life's experiences, but through the minds and hearts of thousands of Dead Saints who have died, been resurrected, and transformed by death's dark door?

In my friends' presence, I realized that my entire life seemed perfectly choreographed in preparation for the writing of The Dead Saints Chronicles.

I shuddered: The cold stone of fate, a pre-set personal "event" or whatever you want to call it, had pounced upon me like a lion. I laid there stunned, its terrible aspect weighing heavy on my soul. Even in this moment of triumph of finishing my research, I was so sad. Not for me, but my family, my friends, and my kids. The odds of such a confluence of events seemed astronomical.

I closed my eyes, "Paul, why did I wait so long to begin? Why didn't I listen?" God had given me signs and dreams for years, like the philharmonic orchestra building its tempo to a final crescendo. Hindsight is 20/20, but the question still begs, "Why did God give me visions of my future knowing I would not decide to act on it before today? Was it a premonition where I could change my destiny, or just a "Get your house in order "vision" and accept the inevitable?"

I sighed and turned to Delynn, "Just fifty more NDE anecdotes from the NDERF.org site to go." Looking back, it's incredible how my NDE research neared completion the night before my surgery, or so I thought. Over the last several months, I had stubbornly persisted through reading and indexing a minimum of fifty near-death experiences a day, out of which I would find ten that merited referencing in *The Dead Saints Chronicles*.

Over the last three years, I had reviewed nearly 5000 near-death testimonials, including reading about one hundred near-death books and Afterlife related studies. It was a typical evening exercise, but I had pushed my research into overdrive now that my life appeared in danger.

It was almost Midnight. I popped that last excerpt in at 11:45 p.m. I turned to Delynn and smiled, "Done! Finally!"

"Way to go, baby!" she whispered. I knew she was almost asleep.

I turned off the light, closed the computer, and set it on the nightstand. We settled to go to sleep. It was late. I closed my eyes to the world and turned to snuggle Delynn. I wasn't tired yet. The Dexamethasone steroids the doctors had prescribed kept me wide awake. I had been able to sleep only a few hours every night.

As I lay there tossing a bit, I imagined what it was going to be like tomorrow when the brain surgeons placed me on the operation table under full anesthesia to take a biopsy of my "brain tumor." Would I have a near-death experience during surgery? What would they find? The live analysis would reveal a virus infection, non-malignant brain tumor, or brain cancer. Either way, I would know the diagnosis and prognosis soon after the surgery was over.

The surgery outcome would impact my life in many ways, but my biggest concern was finishing the books. What if my cognitive functions, my speaking, or my hands' use are impaired? I had so much to do and possibly so little time to do it in, and what I had to do, I had to do it with a melting brain. The weight of finishing the project was overwhelming. The *Chronicles* had become a 1500 single-page document, indexed by subject, but I hadn't started writing the book at all. The *Chronicles* were an indexed reference document. Somehow, I had to integrate my cancer story, weave in the Dead Saint testimonials and write commentaries and theological arguments. Simple, right?

Except for articles I wrote for our church newsletter in the 1980s, I was an unpolished, unpublished author. I had never written a significant book before.

For a moment, I felt a bit like John Carter in Edgar Rice Burroughs's, *The Princess of Mars*. In his worldwide search for a secret alien medallion that would allow him to teleport back to the red planet, he had written down his experiences in a leather-bound manuscript which he passed on with his apparent death to his nephew, Ned. While I was not dead yet, and while the book was not bound in leather rawhide, the Chronicles contained vital information about my revelations about the Afterlife I felt were important to pass on. Published author or not, somehow, someway, I was going to finish this work.

The imaginary ghosts of Paul and Galileo melted slowly into the night. I closed my eyes and tried to sleep. Looking back was difficult. Since January, I felt I had been trying to swim upriver. Nothing was working. I had always imagined myself as a crisp, yellow, fall maple leaf that learned to float down the river of life. If I learned to let myself drift down the river naturally with the steam's current, the maple leaf would only gently cascade by boulders, canyon walls, and rocks.

But the entire last year of my life, I realized I hadn't been floating peacefully along at all. I had been trying to swim upriver, believing I was doing the right thing.

It was a long night. Tomorrow my life was going to change, and I knew it.

~**Dream:** I knew, in my dream, it was Galileo's 449th Birthday. I never tried to calculate the difference in years between his birth on February 15th, 1564, and 2014. The exciting thing is that if you add 449 years to 1564, you get the year 2013. The dream year calculation was off by one year. He was/is 450 years old. Strange. Maybe history has his birth date wrong?

2

The Diagnosis

Early Expiration Date

Swedish Hospital, Seattle, WA, July 1, 2013

I never expected an early expiration date to be stamped on my life.

We awoke in the hotel room the morning of the scheduled surgery at 7:00 a.m. My heart was gently beating and in perfect health, but my mind felt like a shipwreck. Delynn and I didn't speak much. We simply showered, got dressed, and ignored breakfast. I emailed a draft of the book to Delynn just in case something happened. I gazed out of the 8th-floor hotel window one last time, pausing for a moment to soak in the view of the city as it juxtaposed against the granite peaks of the Olympic Mountains towering 8,000 feet over Puget Sound. In early summer, nearly all the snow had melted except for the few white fingers of white near each summit. Still, it's postcard-perfect and breathtaking.

I called down to the valet so they would have our twelve-year-old blue BMW coup warming up and ready to drive when we arrived downstairs. We only had a small, overnight bag to carry on our way down the elevator, but it was mine to carry. Delynn headed to the front desk to checkout, while I stepped outside into the cold morning air to check on the car. Our Beemer was idling at the Hotel entrance, and the tall, friendly Nigerian Bellman already had the passenger door open for me. By doctor's orders, I could not drive because of my brain mass due to seizure threat. I plopped into the passenger seat and waited for her. After forty years of being a "driver," it was awkward being a passenger. It's like being a driver of your own life for forty years, and now suddenly somebody else was in charge of my life. Even though it was my beautiful wife driving, it was still weird.

A few minutes passed before she was sitting next to me, ready to go. As we headed out for the ten-minute drive to Swedish Hospital, I paused to reflect again on what the heck was happening.

July 1st had arrived too soon for any of us. Delynn swerved into the front of Swedish Hospital entrance bringing me back to the present. She likes to drive fast, and today was no different. It was 8:30 a.m. Time to check in for surgery.

The surgeon was going to take up to six match head size samples of the tumor mass in the left hemisphere of my brain. The surgery is not considered high risk, though there is risk of stroke and bleeding with any brain surgery, even death.

We were alone—Delynn and me. No fanfare. No tears. Just a big grin, an in-depth look into the eyes, a kiss goodbye, and I walked off with the RN nurse who brought me down the OR hall to the nearby changing room. I removed my jeans and my cheap $14 Blue Hawaiian Walmart short-sleeved shirt, socks, favorite leather sandals, kept my underwear on (my option), and donned the hospital gown over my nakedness. I put the whole heap in a plastic hospital bag, closed the door behind me, and faced the RN. She helped me up onto the hospital gurney bed, and within five minutes, I had an IV port in my arm and was ready for surgery.

Dr. Ryder Gwinn, my Neuro-Surgeon, right behind her, smiled at me, and reached over with a black indelible ink pen and marked a spot on my left side receding hairline—I guess as a neurosurgeon's dumb safety net to not operate on the wrong side of the brain. X sometimes really marks the spot.

The anesthesiologist arrived to go over the biopsy procedure with me. As they are supposed to do, he asked about my health history, allergies, family health background, which if you have ever been in a hospital, they ask you the same thing at least four times, I guess, for safety reasons.

He asked me what I did for a living, and I went right into my spiel about the writing of the Chronicles and how I had often found anesthesiologists privy to many near-death stories, especially from patients who died on the operation table.

Well, he said, "I've never lost anybody."

"That's good," I thought to myself. "It is too early for a full-blown near-death experience. Not yet. God, there's too much to write about before you take me."

"Mr. Solomon, are you ready?"

"Sure. Let's get it over with."

I was wheeled down a few hallways, through the doors of OR #1, marked by a Sharpie on a white 11x8 sheet of paper.

They wheeled me into a vast futuristic bright white Operation room. Everyone is calm and relaxed. No worries. The Anesthesiologist starts talking to all the OR nurses about my research project on near-death experiences. We were chatting away all of five minutes about the book before putting a breathing mask over my nose and mouth.

It was precisely 9:30 a.m. That was the last thing I remember.

In what seemed like the very next second, the nurse was removing the mask and said, "Ok. Mr. Solomon, how are you feeling?"

It was 1:30 p.m. The biopsy surgery was over.

I had no memory of anything whatsoever, but I was glad everything seemed ok. I was breathing. I felt no pain from the two-inch opening Dr. Gwinn had made in my skull to extract the tiny tumor samples, which he closed up with super-flesh blue. My feet and hands worked. I felt the same way after the surgery as before the surgery.

It was like nothing happened at all.

I turned to my right and saw a patient lying in a hospital bed a few feet away. He was awake after back surgery and told me he was still in a lot of pain.

During my OR recovery, Dr. Gwinn visited Delynn in the Visitor/Family waiting room to go over the surgery results with her. He pulled her aside, and with grim finality, he told her it was his opinion that the 2cm tumor was malignant. Though the results would take about a week to verify, he was sure it was Glioblastoma Multiforme, GBM, type IV.

Delynn looked at the doctor in disbelief, "You mean David has the same cancer my mother had?"

"Yes."

Tears began running down her face. "Really? You've got to be kidding."

"No. I'm pretty certain it's GBM."

She asked, "Have they made any progress in the last twenty years to cure GBM?" He stared at her for a moment in a loud silence, "Not really."

He stared in intense silence, for it seemed to Delynn an eternity. She wanted to hear something different. "They have improved life expectancy maybe to 15-18 months through targeted radiation and chemotherapy."

He took her hand and said, "I'm very sorry, Ms. Solomon." He turned and walked away.

I can imagine it really sucks for a doctor, especially a caring doctor, to bring terrible news to the wife and family. We hadn't expected the cancer to be GBM. Not that. At least something we could fight—nearly 100% fatal killer. There are long term survivors, but you could count them on the one hand.

Back in the OR, I knew nothing of the visitor room news dropped on my wife. God, I wish someone had been there to be with her. We didn't expect it.

Ironically, I felt a bit like Luke Skywalker. The Force ran "strong" in his genetic family because of a power produced by the Midi-chloreans.[2] It occurred in the cells of his father, Darth Vader, and his sister Princess Lea. Still, instead of the life-producing Force, this rare cancer moved through my spiritual family like a lightsaber, cutting through the mitochondria, a necessary component for cells to divide, but in my case, death, not life.

Two people who were a part of my inner circle family died of GBM. My wife's mother, Barbara, age 54 in 1993. My friend, age 55, died of it in 2007. Delynn's dear friend had also died about the same age. At 54, I sit here, wondering. What were the odds that so many in my inner circle would die of the same rare cancer, nearly the same age, and not genetically related?

Astronomical. The coincidences begged an answer. Why did I see my friend die of the same GBM brain tumor in 2007? Why did Delynn's mother die of GBM in 1993? To prepare both of us for my own death from GBM? Was it that simple?

I believe, before we are born, God meticulously plans our birth of our soul, our bonsai tree, its species, the geography where it took root, weather, disease, and strife affecting its shape and appearance, and its

---

[2] A concept created by George Lucas for Star Wars

eventual death. During our bonsai's life, God applies training wires to bend our character's branches in a more beautiful direction by the interaction of parents, family and friends, business, and even tragedy.

3

The Decision

40 Day Journey

Post-Brain Biopsy Surgery, Seattle, WA July 2, 2013

I was reminded of Julianne's, a Dead Saint, "life review," where Jesus told Julianne: *"Fix everything gone wrong. Fix everything that was your fault. DO NOT REMIND ANYONE ELSE WHAT THEY DID."*[3]

A day after the biopsy surgery and after a fairly sleepless night, I awoke with no pain or headaches from the operation. Delynn came in early to the hospital room I was moved to and sat with me through what became a dull day of recovery. She had asked me if the doctor had visited or explained the results of the biopsy. He had not. She waited for hours before deciding it was time to tell me. My children were coming to visit, and she wanted me to know before their arrival. She was the one to share the news. I almost didn't believe it at first. We were both surprised the doctor himself hadn't told me.

Perhaps the good doctor assumed Delynn's experience of her mother's death from GBM twenty years prior would be as good a messenger as anyone. But how can telling your husband that he is going to die be easy? After the initial shock, the news sank in. She had to make phone calls to my mother, family, and friends. The most challenging for her was calling my mother. She first called her daughter to share the dreaded news so she could calm her nerves and shake the shock before calling my mom. She said it was all so surreal. She didn't want to be the one. She was alone.

---

[3] *Julianne D NDE*, #1882, 04.29.09, NDERF.org

We just didn't expect this outcome. The call was finally made. Next would be telling my children when they arrived.

While I lay in the hospital bed, I shared my insights about the book to any passing doctor or nurse who would hear me. Doctors even visited to listen to my story. I was calm about it all. Perhaps I should have read Elisabeth Kübler-Ross' book *On Death and Dying, the five stages of grief*...denial, anger, bargaining, depression, and acceptance. Somehow I jumped right to "acceptance," but at the moment, that's how I felt. Internally I knew my cancer seemed all part of the plan; therefore, a certain excitement prevailed over the fear of leaving my loved ones behind. I would find out later that Ross was right, I would eventually go through the grieving and anger...it would take me time.

Within a few hours around dinnertime, my children and our long-time friend, Stephanie, peeked through the hospital room door holding "Get Well" balloons. They gathered around the end of the bed. I know they were scared. You know, there was always that 'hope the brain tumor would be a blood clot or benign; but that hope was dashed, I think, even before they walked in the room. My daughter Angela had just turned 15 and her brother Ben 18 and were not prepared to handle death, much less the death of their father. I will never forget watching Angela's eyes redden and tear up when I told her the news. She was trying to be so brave. But I could see how scared and how shocked she was. Benjamin was just quiet. He always kept his emotions to himself. I wished he would cry and just get the pain out. Every time I relive this moment, I break down and cry all over again.

I did not want to accept that I would not see Angela turn 18 or see my son have his first real job and gain full independence. It was difficult to accept the hand I'd been dealt. Wasn't there a way for this cup of poison to pass from me?

I wondered if the dreams of Grandma Miller, Paul Solomon, and my precognitions were real. Was I going to die? How much time did I have left? How could I get my life and the *Chronicles* completed in such a short time? How could I effectively write a book with a cancerous brain tumor affecting my thinking? Was my goal just to get my spiritual house in order?

All these questions ran through my mind as I lay there on the hospital bed.

Discharge from Swedish Hospital

I was discharged from Swedish on the 3rd of July with little fanfare and sent home. My follow-up was set for July 12th. I was told I should see a neuro-oncologist to plan my post-surgery treatment strategy. I was on a large number of steroids; I felt invincible, sharing with Delynn all the things I intended to accomplish that day. On our way home, we stopped by the Chinese Buffet to celebrate. I felt disoriented and dizzy, but I still served myself the food from the buffet. As I passed by a mirror, I saw myself for the first time since the biopsy. I realized I had not taken a shower or even washed the gel from the brain biopsy out of my hair. I looked like an unkempt homeless person. I sat down with my sushi and crab legs to eat and looked around the restaurant. I felt like everyone was looking at me. I was officially a person with "cancer," and I knew I would never feel "normal" again. It was more of a shock than the actual biopsy brain surgery.

Since I was taking the high doses of steroids, my mind was on overdrive. I awoke with a start at 3:00 a.m. and began to bang out journal notes. I put together a marketing plan for the *Chronicles,* and I didn't stop until 8:00 a.m. I turned to Delynn and said, "Hun, I want to bring my story to CNN." Perhaps it was just wishful thinking brought on by steroid buzz. I didn't have a dream it would be so.

By 10:00 a.m. I was up and out the door to rid the garden of weeds and do various garden clean-up, including late spring/early summer pruning the dozen twenty-foot Japanese maple trees in the garden.

The weight of "getting our house in order" took on a new meaning.

It was the 4th of July, and throughout the day, friends stopped by for a brief visit; others stayed for my annual fireworks display. Typically, "Dad" was always in charge of fireworks operations, but my inability to "run" away from lit fuses forced me to sit in a lawn chair and watch the show. It was one of my favorite holidays. Ben and his best friend Patrick had the fireworks mantle handed over to them, and they had a "blast" blowing everything up. It's what teenagers like to do.

Dr. Gwinn

On July 12th, we had a follow-up appointment with our neuro-surgeon, Dr. Ryder Gwinn, to go over the biopsy results and look at the next steps, including setting up the resection surgery. He confirmed the diagnosis as GBM. His assessment was slightly optimistic. He discussed the risks and benefits of resectioning the tumor, including the risk of infection, bleeding, seizures, chronic pain, anesthetic risks, stroke, need for re-operation, and other unforeseen complications. Injury to the brain from any of these could produce permanent neurologic damage of almost any type, including sensory, motor, cognitive, or personality dis-functions. He could not answer an array of questions regarding the typical follow-up protocol for chemo and radiation. He said we would need to speak with a neuro-oncologist. Yet, at the time, I felt I understood those risks and wished to proceed with the surgery because that is the typical standard of care for GBM-IV. It is to do surgery and remove as much as the tumor as possible (best results is to take at least 98% of the tumor), then chemo/radiation together for six weeks.

However, he stressed that tumor resection would have a specific risk to my right leg functions, given the tumor's location. He said that an aggressive resection would likely increase my length of survival, but it was highly probable to leave the right side of my body paralyzed, especially my leg and possibly my right hand, which would affect the completion of my book. It weighed heavily on my mind. Though Dr. Gwinn was unable to answer the post-surgery and oncology concerns, we decided to schedule the surgery.

We left the doctor's office with an appointment set for July 26th for a functional MRI and surgery for August 2nd.

As many know, setting appointments, getting approvals from insurance agencies, let alone the Veterans Administration, is a daunting task. The VA approved the outpatient surgery at Swedish Hospital for August 2nd. The VA did not perform this type of surgery. It was frustrating they would not also approve an appointment with a neuro-oncologist. Delynn spent days asking for approval. It fell on death ears.

The VA believed it was standard procedure to do surgery, then chemo and radiation. They failed to realize the type of cancer it was, the type of surgery it was, or the many things to consider. Delynn had dealt with this type of cancer with her mother, so she knew speaking with a neuro-oncologist was extremely important.

Every GBM patient is different, their tumor size, location, age, so many factors go into the decision, and without a neuro-oncologist, we did not feel confident in the process. The VA would not even approve an appointment with their own oncologist. They just didn't feel it was necessary. Delynn, feeling desperate, finally begged to at least see the radiologist. I cannot imagine how an average VET could have gotten all the things required in time before my surgery without a determined advocate as Delynn. An appointment with Dr. Wallner, the radiologist, had been set for the same day as the functional MRI. We went unsure what it would accomplish; maybe we hoped they would give us peace of mind.

Delynn's Dream

The night before my MRI, Delynn had a dream that she had been in a room full of doctors and could see into my brain. She began to argue with the doctors that she saw the tumor empty. It looked like the inside of a wasp nest, but it was empty. She said the tumor is empty! Leave it alone!

Delynn hoped the dream was real. What could it mean? It was very vivid to her. She held her breath through those days, hoping for a miracle.

July 26th, Functional MRI

I spent two hours lying in the MRI machine. I typically get bored, yet this was different because it would use words and sounds, going through speech and eye movement exercises. The functional MRI helps identify the precise location and extent of the mass to minimize the resection amount. After the MRI, we discovered my tumor had already grown 2.5mm to 20mm since June 13th. It's a bizarre feeling, knowing a tumor is growing inside your head.

Dr. Wallner & Dr. Sun

After the MRI, we sat down with Dr. Wallner, and within a few minutes of our conversation, he said, "You know, you don't have to have surgery."

We were incredulous. I looked at him and said, 'Won't I die within a few months if I don't have surgery?'

Without quoting him specifically, the basic conversation went as such: "Well, if you do the "golden therapy" with Temozolomide and radiation, even without the resection, there's only a 10-15% difference in your average life expectancy. So no, you do not have to go through with the resection surgery and risk putting yourself in a wheelchair, and for the quality of life, you say you are seeking an option."

Wow. Our minds were reeling...Delynn's dream, a friend's spiritual insight that I should not go under the knife that would be confirmed by a young man in the medical field. Was that man, Dr. Wallner?

Was this part of it? We both jumped on the suggestion. Really? The odds were that tight? I'd prefer to walk for the remainder of my days. No surgery, no paralysis. When he saw our reaction, I think he was ready to take back what he said. Or perhaps he wondered if he had said the right thing.

We explored the options, and he felt we should meet with another radiologist in the office who was a Fellow at the University of Washington. He thought he might help answer some of our questions as well. An appointment was set later in the day to see Dr. Sun.

Dr. Wallner was genuinely concerned about my life. I shared a little about my Japanese gardens and my book, *the Dead Saints Chronicles*. I found out that Dr. Jeffrey Long, author of *Evidence of the Afterlife*, and founder of the world's largest NDE site, NDERF.org, had preceded Wallner as Radiology's head in Seattle, VA and had relocated to Baton Rouge Louisiana just three months earlier! What were the odds of that?

While waiting to see Dr. Sun, I had to get some blood tests done, and while I was gone, Delynn had gone outside to get some fresh air. She walked by the radiology building and saw Dr. Wallner standing, watering sunflowers, wildflowers, and tomato plants in a small bed of humble soil, surrounded by concrete and buildings. She shouted to him, "How nice to see you watering your garden."

His response was, "Well, I know it is not like David's gardens, but I enjoy it!"

It didn't matter to her; it was a beautiful site— it brought humanness and heart to the situation. It brought a peace that passes all understanding. It was a divine signpost that Dr. Wallner loved "gardening." And maybe we should listen.

We were not done with the day. Before returning for an appointment with Dr. Jason Sun, we had to run off to Sea-tac airport to pick up mom.

The day had become so surreal that I asked Delynn to share her "empty wasp nest" dream about my tumor with Dr. Sun. Why not? She shared it with him, and as you may imagine, he didn't have an "aha" reply, but he did share that a brain tumor MRI image looks like a wasp nest but full of the disease within. It was an "aha" for us. We wondered, were the glia cancer cells going to disappear from the radiation and chemo? Was the dream prophetic, or was it just a hopeful, symbolic wish?

Dr. Sun explained how my brain-cancer was going to be treated. The standard route if we choose surgery would be to wait six weeks for recovery; the approach was five days of high-intensity beams of radiation focused on the tumor and the area around the tumor for five days, combined with an intense five-day chemo-therapy of Temozolomide —one of the only FDA approved cytotoxins approved for GBM. Temozolomide would be taken every 28th day for five days for the next year. After that, we had to get radiation treatments five days a week for the next six weeks. It meant a two-hour round trip drive from Olympia to Seattle for the next six weeks for radiation treatments that took twenty minutes. The doctors didn't want me driving, so the responsibility would fall to Delynn.

My concern was chemo nausea. I didn't want to put my family through more "stuff" if I would die anyway. He reassured me that only 20-30% of GBM cancer patients had severe nausea reactions to the Temozolomide. So if I had a lousy nausea reaction, I could stop the medication. I asked him what side-affects I could expect from the radiation. The most common side-effects were hair loss, short-term memory loss, and extreme fatigue. One of my greatest concerns was writing and how cancer therapy was going to affect my thinking process. It's hard enough to write as it is. I even had a schedule for finishing the Chronicles by the end of October 2013 (ooh, so optimistic).

Dr. Sun mentioned the University of Washington had a Brain Tumor Board who may answer the big question, should I have surgery or not? How could we get the tumor board to schedule a review of my medical records before the surgery scheduled for August 2nd? The Tumor Board only met on Wednesday's. It was already the end of the day, Friday, July 26th. We would need to get all the medical records to them before deciding even to review it. It felt daunting. Yet, Delynn kept my medical records in order and carried them with her for those just in case moments.

Dr. Sun also had reviewed my health records and noted my long-standing relationship with Dr. Lee at the University of Washington. Dr. Lee was in charge of the colitis clinical trial of MLN-001. Perhaps he could influence and encourage the Tumor Board to look at my case on such short notice. I was recovering from the 10:00 a.m. morning meeting with Dr. Waller and shock that I could forgo surgery. Of course, we wanted the brain tumor out of my skull if we could safely remove it.

Delynn faxed the medical records to Dr. Lee's office, went to the MRI department, picked up the MRI images, and dropped them off at UW, while Dr. Sun called the UW Tumor Board. We waited!!

Garden Party & Prayers

We asked our friends if they would help us clean up the gardens during this waiting and decision period before my surgery. The garden party was miraculous. We had people pop in all day, cleaning, weeding, picking, cooking, and shoveling. Many came to pray with us.

The day began with Phil (the Japanese Landscape Master) and many of our local friends, joined our group effort to lay down stone and mulch to pretty up the Japanese maple tree gardens down on the lower half of Akio. The girls worked to clear the overgrown weeds in the vegetable garden and tie up the raspberries, blackberries, and grapes were growing.

We provided lunch, enjoying fellowship with our friends. At one point, Pete suggested we all gather in the living room together to pray for me. Our friends took turns sharing a prayer until it came to my daughter, who had not yet accepted the evidence of God. Scared and angry by the events folding out in front of us, she spoke up and prayed one of the most beautiful prayers I have ever heard:

"God. I haven't prayed like this before, but if you could. please heal my Daddy."

Suddenly we all felt the Presence of God move through the room as she cried out from her heart to the heart of God. Angela had always struggled with her beliefs about God since she was a young child. It was my hope and prayer that she would discover a closer relationship with Christ...maybe this tragedy would help her find a way to know Him.

It was also Delynn's 49th Birthday! We all celebrated, had laughs, tears, and community!

Surgery?

The question went back and forth through my mind like a tennis match. Surgery, no surgery, surgery, no surgery. I didn't know the real risk, so how could I make the right decision? And to be clear, I believed it to be a life and death decision. I knew my children wanted me to stay on this earth longer, even if it meant losing my ability to walk. They wanted me here. Some of my friends cried, "Please do the surgery." They were not ready to see me leave, yet this surgery did not guarantee anything. In the meantime, we waited.

University of Washington Tumor Board

The University of Washington called on July 31st with their review of my brain tumor MRI. Three brain surgeons, each with over twenty-years of brain surgery experience, unanimously recommended NO SURGERY due to the tumor's location and my quality of life concerns.

The board recommendation helped, but I was still unsure. I apprised Dr. Gwinn that we might not go through with the surgery. He said he understood, but he also wanted us to consult with the neuro-oncologist at Swedish Hospital, Dr. Bankers. The VA wouldn't pay for the consult, so we paid for it out of pocket. An appointment was set for Thursday, August 1st, the day before my surgery.

I was thankful my dear friend and fellow pastor, Stephen Haslam, was flying in from Houston, Texas, just in time to be at the meeting along with my mom and Delynn by my side. Stephen has officiated our wedding only two years earlier in Virginia Beach.

Dr. Benkers, what would you do?

Here I was less than 24 hours from surgery, and I was still unsure. My mom, Stephen, Delynn, and I talked about it all during our ride from Olympia to Seattle before our appointment with Dr. Benkers at 4:00 p.m. I was bouncing the pros and cons. Maybe I should still have surgery?

Perhaps I was foolishly risking my life? Would it be better to resign myself to a wheelchair and be able to hug my children? Even that option was not guaranteed. Period What should I do?

Our family team walked into Dr. Benkers' office at Swedish, not knowing what to expect. But the answer was simple. Ask the doctor. What would you do if you were in my position?

So I did. Benkers' responded without hesitation.

She said, "Due to your quality of life concerns, I would not do the surgery. And even if you did choose to go through the surgery and it is safely removed, it could grow back within the six weeks during recovery time. I suggest that you get into radiation therapy and chemo as quickly as possible in hopes to stop the tumor growth."

So that was that. We all looked at each other and said, "Well, that was pretty obvious." The decision now seemed easy. No surgery. At 4:30 p.m., we told Dr. Gwinn's secretary we were canceling the surgery set for 8:30 a.m. the next morning—a surgery only 16 hours away. We set up my first radiation and chemo treatments for August 12th, and that was that.

The drive back home to Olympia was quiet. The weight of making the decision was over. The stress of the moment was gone. Looking back, this was indeed a critical Earth University free-will decision to make. I believe I could count on one hand, fewer decisions that might be just as important as that one.

How did I know it was the right decision? I didn't know. Looking back, it seemed kind of silly that I made the decision such a big deal, but I was intent on making the right decision. I felt everything depended on it. I believe, however, if I looked back at all the major decisions I had to make in my life, most of them still seemed obvious.

Yet, they were my decisions to make. I had to choose. I had to hold onto the steering wheel and "drive my car."

My decision appeared to be the right one. I could still walk, and over the next six weeks of chemo and radiation therapy, this decision would prove miraculous.

Chemo & Radiation Therapy

The day after my decision not to have surgery was a relief, a release, and a let-down. It was like recovering from the shock of a severe car accident. Everyone expected me to go through with the surgery. Instead, we spent the day celebrating, talking, walking in the gardens, picking raspberries, and weeding.

Sarah and Derrick came over to visit. We were still overwhelmed by all the events of the month, and here we were. It was Friday night. Laura and Jim had their weekly Texas Hold 'em poker game. So that night, instead of surgery, we were celebrating with a cash poker game. With the cancellation of surgery, we had decided to move forward with chemotherapy and radiation. Temozolomide (Chemo) and photon radiation therapy were known as the 'golden formula' for treating terminal GBM tumors. My treatment was set to begin on August 12th.

I received last-minute calls from well-meaning friends to go the "natural" route, not to allow the chemo and radiation to have its toll. Or the homeopathy route. Miracle cures from around the world were suggested, including promising stem cell and viral immune therapy. It's all good if you have $100,000 plus for travel and the clinical trials. I read about many GBM cancer patients who spent the last year of their lives chasing after cancer cures—time I could not see was producing results for GBM and was not willing to invest in to save my physical body?

Of course, there were the spiritual healers, the most famous being "John of God" in Brazil who used "spiritual doctors" to perform pretty amazing healings, "cutting" or poking metal surgery devices in the eyeball. Even Oprah Winfrey found him inspiring. No thanks and no offense. Perhaps his healing powers worked for so many, but I just didn't feel it was the right thing to do. My focus was on finishing my books. (In 2020, Delynn heard the news that John of God had been arrested on sexual abuse allegations. Many friends referred me to a doctor in Texas and other clinics throughout the world, but most was tentative at best and "cures" with a price tag starting at $225,000. I was not going to bankrupt our family over a Hail Mary pass.

I was not opposed to going natural but thought it wiser to apply nutritional supplements and diet changes as concurrent therapy. There was no evidence either way, with very few exceptions, that radical nutritional changes had cured GBM. Steve Jobs had been presented with the same choice and still chose radiation and chemo.

What about Homeopathy? Some online brain tumor boards suggested the Banerji Protocol as an adjunct to radiation and chemotherapy. It was inexpensive. It cost only $75 to try taking these tiny white bb sized pills 3x a day. Ruta 6c & Cal Phos (10x) I thought it was a shot in the dark, yet I knew my sister healed herself of Lyme disease using homeopathy. Nearly every European city has a homeopathy clinic on every corner. Unfortunately, it is looked down upon by North America.

I finally ordered the strange round white pills. I only took them for a month before throwing them into the huge basket of vitamins to be retaken someday. I began the Banerji homeopathic therapy again on December 15, 2015, hoping they will help slow down my tumor growth. They are one of the approved, recommended homeopathic GBM therapies on the ClinicalTrials.gov website that effectively reduce brain tumors' size, sometimes eliminating them. Who knew?

I spent a lot of time reading other GBM patients and caregivers' experiences on brain tumor discussion boards, and still do, watching for new treatments and how other GBM patients are coping with the disease.

40 DAYS

As I prepared to make the long drive up to the Seattle VA for my first radiation treatment, I reflected on the spiritual meaning of my 40-day journey since my brain biopsy. There are many references in Biblical tradition using the number 40. It is a number representing a period of spiritual challenge, purification, and testing. Moses was with God on the mount, 40 days and nights (Exodus 24:18). God made Israel wander for 40 years in the wilderness (Numbers 14:33-34). God gave Nineveh 40 days to repent (Jonah 3:4). Jesus fasted 40 days and nights (Matthew 4:2).

Women are pregnant for 40 weeks. The number 40 is also the number for rebirth. The ancient Egyptians believed that the scarab beetle, Khepri, was symbolic of Ra, the rising sun. Just as Ra rolls the sun across the sky, setting in the west rising in the east, the small scarab beetle rolls a ball of dung across the earth. Beetle eggs were incubated in the dung ball for 40 days until the new larva would emerge as full-grown beetles and fly off toward the sun. Thus, the ancient Egyptians began to correlate resurrection with the Scarab.

The 40-day trial after my brain biopsy was an intense period that tested my faith in God and my resolve to complete the *Chronicles*. Did the experience purify my heart? Only God can answer that. Forty days represents a beginning, an ending, and a new beginning again. Growing doesn't stop. Without GBM, I know without a doubt, I would have never written the *Chronicles* because I tended to procrastinate.

Without GBM, I would have never faithfully recorded hundreds of journal notes, dreams, and realizations that occurred during this time about living, death, and the Afterlife. Without GBM, there would have been no pathos, no drama, and no real story to tell. Without GBM, I would not have tried to reconcile many of my relationships. The list goes on and on.

Like the dung beetle, I was emerging from my GBM experience a new and different person, flying towards an unknown sun.

— 4 —

The Dissembling Bonsai Mask

The Beginning – Seeing the Mask
Seattle, Washington

When Delynn and I arrived to begin my first radiation treatment at the Seattle VA Medical Center, I didn't know what to expect.

Dr. Wallner explained how the Gammex Laser System would work. The Multi-Leaf Collimator Device (MLC) and the Modulated Radiation Therapy (IMRT) using the highest radiation required, would bombard the 20mm "octopus" tendrils of the glia-cell tumor directly, without hitting the healthy brain tissue around it.

He said the sessions would only last fifteen minutes. I would feel no burning; however, I should expect significant fatigue after six weeks and that I would lose my hair on one side of my head. (how nice!!)

During my first session, the radiologists measured and fit me with a radiation mask, which holds your head in place while beams of radiation shot through your brain. The plastic mesh is softened with hot water and then applied over the skull and face while hot, which then cools into a hardened form used for the 28 sessions of radiation I would be hit with over the next 41 days. The white tape you see on the side of the mask above is marked with a pen to help align two lasers so that the radiation beams hit their target perfectly – an important safety feature, thank you very much.

An MRI was done to determine how many beams it would take without damaging the brain's vital parts or passing rays through my eyes and the cornea, possibly blinding me. The more beams, the better. The doctors were able to employ seven beams, which was supposed to be a good sign. I would have those beams shot through my skull for five days a week until all 28 sessions were finished. I was also given the chemo cytotoxin pill, Temodar (*Temozolomide*), to take daily for those same six weeks.

As I got to know the radiologists over the next few weeks, I discovered that most of the crew working there knew Dr. Jeffrey Long very well and remembered his studies on near-death experiences. What are the chances of that? There are over 1400 Veteran Hospitals in the US, so it is a strange God breadcrumb indeed that I should be treated at the one place Dr. Long had worked for years.

I had never met Dr. Long, although, of course, I was familiar with his New York Times bestseller, *Evidence of the Afterlife: The Science of Near-Death Experiences,* and his near-death websites. I subsequently discovered he had moved to work at the Baton Rouge, LA, VA Medical Center, as a radiation oncologist there. I eventually contacted him to receive permission to use several hundred quotes from NDE's posted on his NDERF.org website.

What is a radiation treatment like? I'm taken into a room to lie down, having my feet tied and held down, so they do not move, then my mask is slid over my face and clamped into place. There is to be no movement by me. Over fifteen minutes, the radiation machine moves around at different angles, while robotic metal pins changed position within a bright light to redirect the radiation rays. I sometimes drifted off staring into this light and wondered how *many thousand times brighter* the Light must shine in a face-to-face encounter with God, as the Dead Saints so often describe it.

The Mask Metaphor

I wondered about the Mask I wore during therapy as a metaphor in my own life: The mask is symbolic of our personality. It is hardened around our soul, that spark of Light of Heaven, by the time we were six or seven years old. The mask is not the real you. It has been integrated into our body and mind and programmed by the natural settings around us. We think it is who we are, but it is not.

One Dead Saint describes our personality—our Mask, as illustrated in the movie, *The Matrix*. Tim says it is not real:

The information that I received is difficult to put into words as the concept is not applicable in a materialist context. The closest I can come to explaining what it was like is by drawing parallels with the film 'The Matrix' where near the end Neo suddenly sees the computer-generated world for what it is, and realizes just what is real and what isn't, realizes what is lasting and what is temporal, realizes what is important and what doesn't matter anymore.

That's how I felt as if I'd suddenly been shown what it's all about. I felt like I had one foot in this world and the other foot in another one entirely. I'd been given new eyes and could 'see' everything, its temporal nature, how much we emphasize things that aren't that important.

The only thing that matters in this life is where your heart is, who you are, and what kind of person you are. People search for recognition and celebrity status, but it doesn't matter one jot as far as the next life goes.[4]

The Mask: A cardboard shell

In her NDE, Malla was shown a personification of her "created" self that appeared real but was not real. It materialized as a cardboard

---

[4] *Tim E's Probable NDE*, #1347, 12.14.07, NDERF.org

demon that had no individual consciousness. Her cardboard "demon" seemed to have the power of its own to control her life. Even her attempts to "exorcise" the demon through "half-hearted" prayers didn't work to rid her of the darkness. Note the "half-hearted" effort at prayer:

I was presented with a terrifying sight that produced a feeling that literally rattled my whole being. I tried to cover my eyes to avoid looking at what had just unfolded before me, but to no avail. There was no way to avoiding seeing or to hide from that, which is ultimately the reality. At my right, a few feet away, stood something that resembled a demon. It was not your average demon, but one made of cardboard. It looked absolutely ridiculous!

I knew that whatever I was seeing was not real in the sense of being an individual consciousness. It was a product of my own mind. One part of me wanted to laugh at it; another part of me however wanted to scream in terror. I had never imagined a demon made of cardboard before, but it indeed had a terrifying effect on me. 'So, you thought it was that easy, huh?' the demon snarled, as it came bouncing towards me. 'Oh, I know what this is,' I thought. This is my fear manifested: This is my own loathing. This is my lack of appreciation for life and the people in it. This is a learned experience as I walked through life, becoming more and more engulfed in despair. The demon is showing me how I treat myself and others when I am affected by the feeling of fear. This is exactly the tone of voice that belongs to me, when I am being mean towards myself and others. Here it is, manifested as my own personal version of hell. My mind frantically tried to remember one of the prayers I had learned at Sunday school to make the demon go away. After all, that was what I had heard priests do when they expel evil from people, 'Dear Father, you who are in Heaven, your name be holy...!

Peeking through my fingers again, I saw the demon approach closer and closer, seemingly unaffected by my half-hearted effort of praying.

'It doesn't work!' I panicked and screamed with all my might, 'GOD, PLEASE HELP ME!'[5]

Like a bonsai, your "Mask" has form and style. The forces of nature around your tree have hardened its main trunk and branches and set it growing in a particular direction that cannot be changed without making it look "unnatural." Forcefully changing an upright bonsai into a windswept bonsai would "go against its nature." Likewise, we cannot unnaturally change ourselves.

What we can do is accept who we are and make our mask, our Bonsai, more pleasing by pruning and training its branches into a more beautiful form. When Felton Jones, one of my teachers, I share more about him in my first book, pruned my azalea, he did not change the original nature and direction of the tree. He made a space whereby I could grow new branches.

So how do we make our tree more beautiful? How do we remove the mask of our personality to reveal Heaven?

The shaping of the mask comes in many different forms.

Radiation treatments became a boring daily 120-mile, round-trip nightmare, just to go through a 15-minute radiation therapy session. On our first trip up to Seattle, Delynn landed a speeding ticket.

Between the radiation treatments, we had been selling everything we could to raise cash; my 3500 Dodge Ram Truck, (cry, cry) our 40 foot, 1971 Cruise a Home, stocks, and artwork. Everything always seemed to sell "just in time" to pay our monthly bills.

---

[5] Malla Possible NDE/STE, #3933, 04.27.15, NDERF.org

I had to make so many decisions, including selling my beloved home. Forty days prior, I had imagined that I would die looking up at the Sistine Chapel painting of God reaching out to touch Adam's finger on my ceiling in my home. Even though I was determined to die in my home, it was looking less and less probable, with monthly bills and mortgage going unpaid if we waited out the cancer for more than six months—a tactic that would likely end in bankruptcy and a forced repossession of the house.

August was a blur. I was coming to the realization my life was dramatically changing. I spent my days working in the gardens. It was my peace, my solitude, my communication with God. How much time did I have at Akio?

Being terminally ill was hard on Ben and Angela. July and August were incredibly hard on both of them. All our family's past issues came up. Angela was angry, especially since I had so quickly resolved myself to dying. Without realizing it, my acceptance of my death only stirred anger in her. She thought I was ok leaving her. She was hurt and afraid.

Angela flew to Virginia Beach for the yearly visit to see family. It was the first time I had not gone with my kids to Virginia Beach. We had an incident that happened during her stay, which I placed several "restrictions," causing Angela to react so violently, speaking harsh words to me. Though I understood she was having a difficult time with her mother and dealing with my cancer diagnosis, it broke my heart that I thought I would never recover. She didn't want to return. She asked if she could stay with my sister, with whom she was very close.

She did return home at the end of the visit to more turbulent times. I was becoming increasingly weak, losing my hair, swollen from steroids. And I was now considering selling the home that had been Angela's since she was seven.

Some long-term relationships began to fall apart, including my dad, who stopped talking to me. Delynn and I were challenged by gossip that I had an affair on her the year earlier; that we were hiding money and telling people we were broke for sympathy; and that I was wrong not to do surgery to extend my life. It was exhausting. I wanted to reconcile all of my relationships. I wanted to be at peace with everybody, yet a more significant divide was happening.

I was so weak and tired; I felt I had given so much to those relationships, and still, to this day, I do not understand what happened. I often joke to Delynn that I will have to wait for the Life Review to understand the dynamics.

August 20, 2013, Delynn and I celebrated our second wedding anniversary at a local steakhouse restaurant (Richardo's in Lacey, WA) with fine red wine and ribeye steaks. I remember thinking my mother lost her second husband during their second year of marriage. He was the love of her life, as Delynn was mine. Was family history repeating itself?

By the end of August, I had my attorney update my Will and create a Trust for the children. She suggested I do whatever it took to have my things in order and not leave it to Delynn to carry on after I was gone.

We finally made the decision to sell the house and Akio Gardens. I knew we would take a significant loss selling, having invested over $800,000 in the gardens alone. I knew I would never get back all the money I had put into it, let alone my blood, sweat, tears, and love I had committed.

I felt I was losing everything.

The question was, could we sell Akio? How long would it take? The sale would pay off all our debt and get the monkey off our backs. And then what? Where would we move? Should we stay in Olympia, rent an apartment and be near my kids, or move somewhere else? Delynn suggested the possibility of moving to Virginia Beach because my Mother, sisters, and family would be there to support us when my health deteriorated. It seemed like a logical conclusion.

We assumed it would take at least six months to a year to sell and had it in our minds that we would move to Virginia Beach the following summer, hoping to take Angela and Ben if he wanted, with us.

Sometimes, when we seek God's direction and don't know the answer but make a move in faith, the doors open, and you know you are doing precisely what you are supposed to be doing.

Akio sells in less than 24 hours!

When major decisions are based on the fact you've been given an expiration date, you become keenly aware of everything, hoping your choices are right. Never really knowing, but following the doors that open. Once the decision was made to sell the house, everything happened so fast. Too fast for all of us to have comprehended, yet the doors opened, and we walked through them.

A realtor was selected, a decision and story within itself. Our realtor, Nancy, had a buyer within 24 hrs. Not only did the buyer want the house, but they also wanted all the furniture, the artwork, the garden tools, the tractor, and, most of all, my beautiful bonsais! Wow, we did not have to go through the painstaking process of selling everything, having an estate sale, or sending our art to a broker. The buyer bought everything we did not keep.

Now what! Facing a beautiful miracle, yet this was not in our plan, we were not expecting to make a move now! We didn't have time to process it all, yet here we were.

A break from radiation, off to Victoria, Canada

It was a gorgeous, sunny September Labor Day. We needed a break from the radiation treatments, so instead of making the long drive back to Olympia, we took the Coho, V.M Ferry from Port Townsend to Victoria, Canada, and stayed in a hotel there. On the ferry over to Vancouver, we sat next to a family who had recently lost a loved one and began talking about life after death. The Coho had a bookstore, and strangely enough, had the bestselling books, *Proof of Heaven* and *Heaven is for Real*. I bought a copy of each for the family, who was surprised and grateful.

We soon arrived and docked at the Vancouver port late that afternoon. The hotel was only a few blocks from the port, and we didn't want to pay for a taxi, so I gutted it out and made it just fine. After checking in, we ate dinner at a restaurant around the corner. Delynn saw there was a Victoria Ghost tour, so we made reservations. Of course, it was a night tour and to me felt hokey—a walking tour which I dreaded. Starting, we didn't know it would be a two-mile exploration of the 1880s of downtown Victoria, all very interesting, but for me, I felt like I was stumbling through a nightmare. I didn't let Delynn how I was feeling, but she knew the tour was too long. I was very, very tired. I took a 200mg caffeine capsule to help me get through the night. Things had changed for me.

We took the V.M Coho back to Port Townsend the next day and stayed overnight there.

We had another treatment on Monday, September 8th. It was the 15th of 28 scheduled radiation treatments. Half-way done. So the doctors were right; during week three, I began to feel "bone-tired." I still feel like I've had a dozen drinks without the benefit of feeling good. Just disoriented and unfocused all the time.

Sometimes, I just wanted to die and get it over with, but it seemed every day I was reminded that someone would benefit from my story and research. I have to get through this therapy and finish the Chronicles. David, press on. Don't give up. Maybe after the radiation is done, my brain will heal a bit, and I will be more focused.

At least, that was my hope.

I was becoming more fatigued from the chemo and radiation as the days went on. With the decision made to sell Akio, we were on a fast track to getting the house ready for sale. We hired a few more contractors to help spiff up the place, including filling in the 220,000-gallon Japanese Coy pond on the lower part of the gardens, we had spent thousands of dollars to dig out.

Ben and his friend, Nathan, worked non-stop cleaning up and weeding the gardens. I had purchased 31 bare root Japanese Akebono flowering Cherry Trees the previous spring in plastic pots, which needed to be planted along the lower driveway. I had bought them before my illness but felt compelled to plant them as my finishing touch to my Akio. She was my baby. I wanted her to bloom after I was gone. In ten-years they would be spectacular. I wanted at least that part of my garden vision realized.

Attack of the Yellow Jackets!

I never liked bees, especially hornets and yellow jackets. Bees were only one of two things I feared. I was always amazed by honey bee fanatics could have their bodies covered with honey bees and not get stung. How brave.

However, I guess yellow jackets were another story; as for my other "fear," you will have to wait and read it about it later. Like a Japanese garden, you can't show everything at once.

Anyway, we were all doing our part to clean up the property. At the bottom of the hill, I was alone picking up debris when I pulled an empty old 5-gallon plastic pot out of the ground. Suddenly I had yellow jackets swarming everywhere. Luckily, I had my Apollo 13 *"Failure is not an Option"* long sleeve hoodie and rubber gloves. I had lived there ten years and had never run into a ground nest of yellow jackets this size—and certainly not one that would attack me!

Anyone can tell you when a swarm of bee's attack, you RUN. It was 600 feet, up a 15% incline, to the top of the hill to the safety of my home. I am not one to be afraid, but I knew if I did not get to the top of the hill and into the safety of the house, I would be killed. My survival instincts kicked in. I was afraid.

I was already wobbly, and my equilibrium off because of the tumor and surgery. So I ran uphill, falling every ten feet, yelling "help!" simultaneously. It was a survival instinct, but looking back, I almost watched myself run up the driveway in 3rd person. Initially, I reached the top of the hill, ran into the garage out of breath, barely croaking out "bees!" Delynn and Benjamin finally heard me, but I didn't stop moving. I ran into the house with them swarming, slamming the door behind me.

Following me, Delynn and Ben stripped off my clothes and swatted all the bees off of me. I had at least twenty bee stings. Both Delynn and Ben were stung several times. We found bees crawling around for days afterward.

A few days later, we ordered an exterminator to come out to our property and kill the bee nest in the ground. I was amazed that he could stand only ten feet away from them without being stung. I asked him, "What is your secret?"

He said, "yellow jackets follow the noise. That's why they followed you."

Earth University note: *When bees attack. Be silent. Don't yell, but be ready to run.*

Last radiation treatment: September 23, 2013

I remember two things, the radiation doctors gave my mask back to me to take home as a memory, and second, Delynn got a speeding ticket driving back to Olympia. When I got home, I thought about keeping the mask—which seemed morbid. I did not want to be reminded of the experience. So without too much thought, I threw the Mask and my old personality in the garbage.

~Zen Masters call our spiritual journey to find our True Self "The face we had before we were born." In like manner, the Japanese have a saying, "Evil is good with a mask on." Remember the Star Wars story of Darth Vader when Luke told his father, "I know there is still good in you." The real you is the good inside of you. The Greeks had it right when they used the word Hypocrite, meaning "actor." Like Darth Vader, who removed his "mask," we are often hypocrites playing a role, wearing a mask, rather than being "real."

A Dead Saint or anyone has the potential to drop the façade of the "Mask." Even after an NDE or transformational experience. The Saints don't protect the mask—they just know it's there. They can no longer delude themselves about immortality or the existence of life after death, and often even the knowledge that the Source of Life—God—exists. The Saint no longer feels the need to project an "I" to protect themselves.

The Holy Fool is the one who drops the mask. Consider Saint Francis, who unrobed himself "naked and clean before God" in front of his village. Planting the "I am saved" button in our hearts is just a beginning point for our spiritual growth. ~**David Solomon, Chronicle 426**

5

The Departing
Garden of Cowboy "Job"

~November 5, 2013. The intensity of leaving Akio gardens finally hit me the week before we were scheduled to leave. I was bald. I shaved my head because the chemo and radiation caused most of my hair to fall out. I always liked my hair, but now it was gone.

I truly felt like Job in the Bible, who lost his health, wealth, and family. Job was written as a parable, given of God, to the Sons of God. The story illustrates a challenge from Satan who said to God, and I paraphrase, "~ not being fair with me because you put a fence around Job I can't get through to tempt him as I would. Now, if you could let down that fence a little bit, that I might get through and present temptation before him, then I could get to him with temptation, and he would be led astray. And being led astray, it would show he doesn't love you, does he?"

God answered and said to Satan, "Do what you will with him, for I have given him strength. He is a man of God. Place your temptation before him and see if he will be led astray. I will allow only one thing: that you will not be allowed to pluck him out of my hand. He may be tempted as a man of God."

The parable was written for all of us. You can see yourself in this situation, as it was later written in the Book of Isaiah, "Will God then allow the evil one to tempt you, to take you away, snatched from the hand of God?" Will a mother leave her suckling child?"

But when you are in the midst of pain, suffering, and loss, it's hard to remember the lesson of Job and God's promises. I found myself emotionally alone and confused. Like Job, whose three friends verbally persecuted him, I later lost three friends.

Job himself did not understand why the tragedy happened to someone who had such great faith in God. Why was a good God allowing such terrible things to happen to a decent, God-loving human being? Job, in short, is asking, "Why me, Lord?"

I asked God the same thing. Why? Why end my life now? I had dedicated these gardens to you. Why are you taking them away from me? Selling my Dodge Ram 3500 truck, my tractor, and my wife sold her guns. (That's the cowboy part! ☺). I was leaving Ben to be on his own in Tacoma, and I was leaving Angela to live with her mother. In some ways, I felt I was abandoning them. Or was God taking them away?

Through his agony, Job became increasingly confused, perplexed, discouraged, without hope. In his worst nightmare, Job sees death coming around the corner of his life, ready to run him down. Job knows he is finished — through. He sees himself doomed to die a broken, lonely, hated, and despised person. Job's hopelessness is painted throughout the book. In one place, he moans, *"My spirit is broken, my days are cut short, the grave awaits me"* (Job 17:1)

Like Job, I had resigned myself I was going to die. My grave was waiting for me. I was not afraid, but my fate appeared inevitable.

In the garden, raspberries were still on the vine. I would lose them too. In my mind, I went through every corner of the garden I loved so much; the crunch of the gravel under my feet; the red color of the Japanese maples, the bright green moss growing in the strolling garden, the rhododendrons that would bloom yellow, red and pink in the spring. The Japanese fence, stained in dark brown, nearly a quarter-mile in length, and designed with yin and yang bamboo that surrounded Akio like a prayer that said, "*This is the Lord's place. Please walk here in peace*," and the thick green bamboo forest that lined our north fence; I remembered every tree we cut and trimmed; every granite stone we placed; every walkway stone laid; the water tsukubai, where so many species of birds washed and drank every morning; and the pine that shaded them.

I remembered the red azaleas blooming and the dozen little gardens no one noticed. I had begun training three different colored varieties of wisteria up the brick facing of the house. I remembered all these beautiful memories. I also remember the hard-to-do chores, like weeding the millions of weeds growing in the moss, but I also recall all the lessons I learned while weeding; the more you weed, the more weeds appear—everywhere magically. Young weeds are easier to pull than old ones. Old weeds have deep roots, and younger weeds are more numerous. Weeding helps focus the mind; it quiets the mind. It enables you to organize. Weeding also attracts friends who want to weed with you, and friends who weed with you don't talk while weeding.

The hard things included splitting 15 cords of wood with my best friend, David, and my Dad, and (literally) the thousand tons of stone we hand-carried from spot to spot. I remembered all my friends and family, who were the wind beneath my wings, who were hardly ever noticed, Phil, David B, Scott and John, Mike, Saint Rick, Ron and his staff, and my loving children, Benjamin and Angela.

And Delynn, who inspired me, loved me, and most of all, walked beside me from the very beginning to the bitter end of Akio. She was losing her beautiful home, a place of refuge, a house of healing, and entertainment. Our home, where Christmas parties were a catered annual event lined with torches up the driveway. That would be gone too.

I may have been a fool with some of the money; nevertheless, I had lost my wealth in building Akio Gardens, the money I could not recover when I sold my property. I lost my dream. I was leaving my kids and my father. My bonsai trees, friends now in the hands of a new caretaker, and my trees were like children to me. I was leaving them too. It was a beautiful dream, but in a week, it would no longer be mine. There was no last-minute rescue coming.

God and the universe were still converging on November 12, 2013, our departure date, and there was nothing I could do to change or stop it. The yellow leaf floating down river didn't seem like a gentle stream right now. It was more like a raging river, and I just had to flow with it.

On November 10, two days before our departure, I held a bonsai class for the new owner, his gardeners, and a few friends, including Sarah. She inherited a century-old excellent Juniper bonsai from me. Even though the time of year was not best for repotting and trimming roots, we repotted two bonsai and spent time with a small paintbrush painting the exposed dead trunk (called *Jin*) of a few trees with sulfur, which turns in a few hours, white. It was a great class.

On November 11th, I drove Angela to her school for the last time. It was awful. Was I doing the right thing? I could hardly keep it together. Tomorrow was coming too fast. We had nothing to sleep on because the furniture was all packed, so we stayed at a friend's house. I took a sleeping pill and crashed.

The next day November 12, we arrived early to prepare for our walkthrough of the house and gardens with the new owner at 10:00 a.m. Before they came, I had to go by the Post Office to mail a few boxes to the cable company, pick up my coffee, and say goodbye to Shelly and Chrissie, the convenience store clerks, always smiled at me and continued contacting me about my health, even to this day.

On my ten-minute drive back to Akio, I don't know if the stress of the moment caused it, but I soiled myself on the way back from the store. I still had colon issues from time to time, but this was the worst bowel accident ever, with crap running down my legs to my shoes. It was awful. In tears, I called Delynn, telling her I didn't know what to do. The new owner was waiting to go through the house and walk the property, and I was already 15 minutes late.

She let the owner know that I had to take care of a "few things" when I got back. I quietly slipped by him, walked stiffly upstairs, and, as much as I could, tried to act as nothing had happened. Upstairs, I stood there in tears while Delynn stripped off my horrible, stinking clothes —black Coho Sweater and new jeans and stuffed them in the garbage and threw them away.

Now I was bald, covered in shit, and still had a brain tumor.

I took a quick shower to clean myself up. I do not know what I would have done if Delynn were not there to assist me. I don't think I ever felt so humiliated in my entire life. I asked God again, "Why? Why are you doing this to me?" It was nearly the final Job "straw" that broke me in half. I didn't get mad at God; I just wanted to know "why?" I've lost my friends, my home, my garden, my dream, my kids, my wealth, and my health. What did I do to deserve this?

In the Biblical story, Job could only assume God was persecuting him. He lashes out at God in pain and anguish. "If I have sinned, what have I done to you, O watcher of men? Why have you made me your target?" Job complains (Job 7:20)

It wasn't that Job had to overcome a specific sin, but rather that he had to grow in understanding. After a lengthy trial, Job eventually hears God's argument about all the good things in the universe, to which Job responds: "I despise myself and repent in dust and ashes" (Job 42:6).

But repent of what? Of some specific sin? Not quite. Job explains, "Surely, I spoke of things I did not understand, things too wonderful for me to know."

I guess, too, there are many things I still do not understand, and I do not know. Yet, God is merciful. I later came to understand "why" this tragic path had befallen me, not because I am wise, but because he allowed me to turn lead into gold and use this horrible experience to become a beautiful lesson for many in writing the *Chronicles*.

I had to take a moment to breathe.

I was now clean, changed, and had new clothes. Any further debate with God would have to wait until we are driving down the road in a few hours. The owner and his staff were waiting.

I came downstairs, business-like. I proceeded with the property walkthrough as if nothing happened. I walked through all five acres of Akio, noting all three water irrigation systems, all trees needing particular care, checking the water well-head locations, water cutoff valves. I looked at the tulips, the vegetable gardens, and all the pruning that should be done to the white pines and Japanese Maples. It's difficult to stop talking about the garden you love.

Be sure to water the Cherry trees.

Divide the tulips every two years.

Fertilize the gardens twice a year.

I conveyed to the garden caretaker that the purple magnolia next to the Zen wall had hundreds of buds that would flower in the spring. Last year, after transplanting the tree, only ten buds bloomed. I could only imagine how beautiful it would be next spring.

Then the walkthrough was over. It was time to leave. Jim, the new owner, helped load our luggage in the trunk of our white Hyundai. I gently filled the empty back seat with three bonsai not sold to the owner.

We were ready to go.

Leaving Akio for the last time

We waved goodbye and slowly drove down the gravel driveway, past the ten-ton granite stones that bordered Akio's hillside, the *Akibono* flowering cherry trees, and the fall yellow and red of the Japanese maples below, and through the walled entrance of my beautiful garden.

In a blink, we turned right and drove to the end of the street, and made our final right turn onto the main road. Just as we turned, a SOLITARY WHITE BALD EAGLE immediately circled over the car at treetop level, wings full spread—both Delynn and burst out crying because it was like an electric shock that passed through us. I had heard eagles by their cry over Akio before but had never seen one fly over our home. The beautiful bird continued to circle overhead. It was like God says in Isaiah 40:31, "But they that wait upon the Lord will renew their strength they will mount up as eagles. They will run and not be weary; they will walk and not faint."

An hour before I was in despair, an hour later, the Eagle helped renew my faith. God was with us, and I knew without a doubt, all was well with God and me. I am sure it always was. I knew we were heading in the right direction.

Tibetan monks have a fascinating discipline of creating a beautiful work of art by coloring sand and then spending days, weeks, and sometimes months meticulously scraping the sand granules through a narrow, metal tube onto a framework of art, resulting in a spectacular, detailed, masterpiece, – and then, with no attachment, it is ritualistically swept away with a brush into a jar, wrapped in silk, and transported to a river where it is ceremoniously released.

I realized *Akio was my sand mandala.*

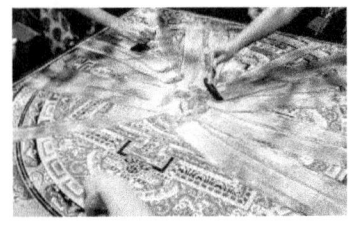

Nothing is permanent in this world. Sometimes our lives have to be shaken up, changed and rearranged to relocate us where we're meant to be. I had to let Akio go.

It was a beautiful sunny day as we began our long three-thousand-mile trek towards Virginia Beach. Delynn and I looked at each other through our tears, and without a word, drove straight on.

~Delynn and I returned to visit Akio in July 2015. We had a two-hour visit to Akio with the kids, Sarah, Rick, Mike, and Achala. It was the first time I had seen them in nearly two years. Any past issues between us seemed wholly healed. Rick was still a smoking chatterbox, but that's why I like him! Jim made a few great additions to the property. He installed an iron gate/security system and paved the upper driveway. The entire two-hour visit was surreal. Delynn and I feel strangely disconnected from it all. Everything. Of course, I am interested in seeing the property "move on," and I am happy Jim is the owner. He has four giant dogs and his kids, who are the same age as Benjamin and Angela were when we moved there.

Now, he just needs a Japanese gardener to apply good pruning! Attachments come in all forms. Even Akio. **~Chronicle 754**

─── 6 ───

The Distance

Take Me Home Country Roads

~Drive from Olympia, WA to Virginia Beach, VA.
November 12, 2013. Chronicle 152
I looked at the three bonsai trees bouncing gently in the backseat of our Sonata as Delynn drove 80 mph down I-5. The Juniper was dying from spider mite infestation. Even though I had sprayed it with spider mite killer, it seemed to be a lost cause, like me and my brain cancer. It seemed inevitable. Why bother to save us if we were going to die anyway?

I closed my eyes for ten minutes to breathe in everything that had just happened since departing Akio. A grown man sitting in a passenger seat, letting a woman drive this fast, is just not normal. Closing my eyes to "trust" her was more problematic than trusting God, not because she was a lousy driver, but because she entertained herself with Facebook on her smartphone while driving. I had to trust that we would not run smack into a tractor-trailer while my eyes were closed. I almost felt like I was her Facebook guardian angel or something like that.

I was getting better at letting go, so as I said, my eyes were closed. It was the fifth time I was making the driving trek across the country; this time, however, I believe it would somehow be my last.

No control. Whatever God wanted me to do, I was His to move around like a pawn in a chess game. The current, God's current, pulling the maple leaf onward down-stream, around rocks, boulders, sometimes faster, sometimes slower, through ravines, over waterfalls, sometimes gets stuck in a log jam; sometimes barely moves along gentle current for many days and weeks.

The yellow leaf-flowing-downriver analogy seemed important. When we have an essential decision to make, how do we know we are making the right decision to turn right or left? Do we have free will to choose? Or are we fated to live out our lives like a puppet with no choice in the matter? If life is entirely at the mercy of fate, then how do we find Heaven? Those who are born into tragedy, who grow up in war-torn families; who have lives of pleasure and wealth versus those born into abject poverty? Is Heaven a one-shot pony? If you miss Heaven, as they say, is it merely too bad? Why would God have 4.8 billion other souls born into a country, family, and religion where they would not get to know Jesus directly or would likely reject Him because of the circumstances in which they were born?

I had traveled the world for a decade and had in-depth spiritual discussions with people of many faiths; Jewish, Muslim, Hindu, Buddhist, Shinto, American Indian, Egyptian, Zoroastrian. I think God allows people to choose their path up the sacred mountain and does NOT judge their right to enter Heaven except by the *love in their hearts*.

I remembered watching a nine-minute video on YouTube of Afshin Yavid, a Muslim man in prison, who cried out to Allah for help and asked forgiveness for being a bad Muslim. A story told in *the Dead Saints Chronicles, a Zen Journey through the Christian Afterlife* in chapter 24, I mention it briefly here to make a point. He cried out from the depth of his soul. Jesus appeared to him in his jail cell in a brilliant white light. It was a powerful, wonderful, life-changing mystical experience. No scripture. No judgment. Just a face-to-face encounter with Jesus, our Planetary Headmaster.

And even though Islam teaches "God has no Son," he is now a Muslim who believes *Jesus is the Living God*. And I suspect he still believes there is no conflict between Islam's teaching that "God has no Son" and Christianity after meeting Jesus Christ, who told him He was the Living God. It is his unique perspective. His conversion to Christianity had nothing to do with religion. It had to do with a direct encounter with the Being of Light, Jesus Christ.

Sighhh. I always rooted for the underdog—especially those who have left the church, disgusted with the fearful punishment theology they endured as children.

I listened to my cousins' husband's tearful story one evening talking about his childhood's punishing religion. His family attended church five times a week, including tent rivals. The Gospel was pounded into his soul at all times. "Save the Sinner," "Bring them to Jesus, lest they go to Hell for eternity." At home, his father repeatedly whipped them, quoting Scripture during the frequent beatings. He remembered secretly wishing his father would die.

Three hundred days of church gospel every year, threatening damnation wounded his soul. He is an exceptionally good man, yet he will not go near a church. To be fair, many pastors, priests, ministers have begun to turn the corner towards teaching love in the church and dropping the sword of punishment. Yet, I believe Jesus is still too often used as a battering ram to push narrow beliefs upon us rather than introducing Christ as an infinite, gentle, forgiving, loving, transforming Lamb he truly is.

My last four years of Dead Saint studies revealed no exceptions to the Heavenly reality of a Loving, non-judgmental God. And more than that, Heaven was not an exclusive club for one religion.

I always looked forward to traveling across the country. I remember when I helped a friend move his furniture and belongings in a 26 foot U-Haul across the country from Nashville. He could not make the trip because of a painful back injury, so I volunteered to be alone on the long journey to think and write.

Here I was again with a lot of time to reflect on my past. I opened my eyes, relieved we hadn't hit anything, opened our CD holder, picked out a John Denver CD, and pushed it into the CD player.

"Almost Heaven, West Virginia. Blue Ridge Mountains, Shenandoah River. Take me Home Country Roads to the place I belong..." played, and in moments I was onion eyed again—or in the Japanese vernacular, "wasabi eyed."

The forces that shaped my life were taking me home, home to my family, mother, sisters, and spiritual family.

But first, I had one more stop.

Saying Goodbye to Dad

Before I knew it, we had driven 90 miles down I-5 and were taking the Kelso exit. Within minutes we quickly arrived at my Dad's home and parked in the driveway.

My visit with Dad and his wife, Lou, was awkward.

My Dad and my mother divorced in 1979, and he had relocated to the West Coast and remarried. I rarely spoke with Dad or saw him until I moved to Washington State in 1995. In 1997, I asked him to join my company, Fast Transact, as a sales agent. He was a natural, and he did very well, receiving monthly residual income for nearly a dozen years. I made Dad part-owner and a director on the company Board.

When we sold the company on January 31, 2010, Dad reaped the benefits too.

After Dad's third wife, Nancy died of ALS in 2009 after 15 years of marriage, Dad met Lou six months later and married. His second wife had also died. Lou and I never seemed to connect. So, as I was saying, our visit to Kelso was awkward. I was still bald from radiation and wore my Harley bandana. Perhaps I was too casual talking about death and my terminal illness. I am not sure. How would I say goodbye, knowing I might not ever see my Dad again? We chit chatted for an hour, but soon the atmosphere in the room became a bit uncomfortable. It was time to go. "Well, Dad, we have a long trip ahead of us, and we want to reach Pendleton, Oregon, tonight."

Dad had told me that he would not have the money to fly out and see me when I died. The moment was befuddled. When we sold Akio and paid off all our debt, he had expressed a need for his financial situation, yet we had just enough money to make a move and live another 12 months, my expected maximum life expectancy.

We hugged each other, and I said, "*Dad, I will see you on the other side....*" not a particularly nice thing to say, but it's what popped out of my mouth. I didn't know what else to say. As we drove away, I felt he was hurt, not by what I said, but by something I did not do. Dad had wanted something from me that I could not give him, maybe it was the money, but it felt more profound than that. I knew there was an issue we needed to resolve, but I couldn't at *that moment fix it.*

The hardest thing about saying goodbyes are all the things I didn't say, all the unresolved stuff, and hurt feelings. I wanted to heal them. I also discovered I couldn't if the other person refused to help in the healing process.

Since November 13, 2013, Dad and I have not spoken. Today is February 13, 2016, the last day edits were completed for the book, but I did find out Dad had sold his house and moved to the Northeast.

At least he is close by when my time comes. I have instructed my family to contact Dad to drive down and see me near death. I pray he comes. *He did not come, but he and David talked just before David's passing.

Cross Country to VB and beyond....

November 12, 2013, Cross County Trek to VB, The Dalles, Oregon

Hwy 84 cuts and snakes its way along the Columbia River through the Cascade Mountains dividing Oregon and Washington State. Five thousand-foot cliffs border each side of the grand gorge, occasionally broken by breathtaking waterfalls cascading down.

Late November snow and ice and wind through the Gorge can sometimes be awful, but we were in luck. Clear, cold weather predominated, allowing us to arrive in Pendleton sometime before midnight.

We stopped at The Dalles to eat a great seafood dinner (fish and mussels) in the late 19th century Baldwin Saloon. On our way to Pendleton, Oregon, we gassed up at a convenience store and picked up a Bald Eagle shirt and a Bald Eagle hat to reflect the Bald Eagle God sent us as a parting gift. Leaving Washington State had come full circle. I had moved to Washington from Virginia Beach in 1995, nineteen years ago.

As we drove across the state line to Oregon, I realized I would never be going this way alive again. ~**Chronicle 152**

November 14, 2013, Cross County Trek to VB. Salt Lake City, Utah

First light, we drove towards Salt Lake City and went straight through, hoping to reach the Mormon City by dinner-time. We had dinner with Richard Davis, a long-time friend in the payment industry. I left that evening, knowing I would not see Richard again.

The next morning, we visited the Mormon Temple and toured it with Sandra, our close friend. Cheyanne, Wyoming, a long 6-hour drive.

The visit to Salt Lake reminded me of a memory that happened twenty years earlier in 1994. While living in Virginia Beach, I had a gut feeling I should move to Salt Lake City to take advantage of a business opportunity. While I can use the excuse that my business idea whisked my family away to Utah, and eventually to Washington State, the truth of the matter is I was running away from carrying any responsibility as Paul's Apprentice and Adopted Son. I believed that I had heard everything spiritual a human could absorb. I was done with it. Not only did I leave Virginia Beach, but I also left any commitment to the Gospel ministry behind and, in many ways, turned my back on that Living Presence, who I had formerly known so well. So now you know the rest of the story. ~**Chronicle 154**

November 15, 2013, Cross County Trek to VB. Cheyanne, Wyoming

At first light, we drove onward towards Wyoming, a vast expanse that looked like a nuclear blast hit it. You can see for a hundred miles. We rolled into Cheyanne, Wyoming, about 4:00 p.m. and looked for the oldest Hotel in town, and found the Wrangler. Delynn and I adore old hotels, and this one was at least a hundred years old, so it qualified. Creaky oak wood floors covered each floor. We chose a room at the far end of the Wrangler, hoping for some privacy. We were tired from the long drive and needed to eat. I remember the shrimp and fish we ordered (why we ordered seafood in perhaps the biggest steak state in the Union I will never know), but it was one of the better seafood dinners I had eaten in a while. Wrangler notes: The view was of a brick wall, and the mattresses were hard. A historical hotel is sometimes not the best place to get a good night's sleep. ~**Chronicle 155**

November 17, 2013, Cross County Trek to VB. Kansas City, Mo.

I began lowering the steroid, Dexamethasone from 4mg a day to 3mg a day on November 18th; 2mg on Nov 19th; 1mg on November 23rd.

Doctors later told me I could have killed myself, lowering the Dex too fast. I became so lethargic, unbalanced, and wonky; I thought I was dying. Maybe that's why my hard drive crashed. Techs call it the "Blue screen of death." So much for using a computer to work on *The Chronicles* for the rest of the trip to Virginia Beach. Uggh.

We stayed overnight with Jacky, one of Delynn's dearest friends in Missouri. Jacky had once prayed "passionately" for me over the phone a few months back after discovering my cancer. I felt the "heat" of her prayer drip over me like warm honey. It was the most intense, heartfelt prayer I had ever experienced. Jacky's mother, who had come to visit while I was there, felt like a sister to me – a warm Christian woman who I seemed to know somehow, but whom I had never met. We were halfway through the trip, but I became so tired, fatigued, weak, sick from the change in medication that we decided to cut the cross country safari shorter than we planned. ~**Chronicle 157**

November 18, 2013, Cross County Trek to VB. Nashville, TN

We rolled into Nashville, Tennessee, late that night. It was Delynn's hometown of Honky Tonkin, but it wasn't the plan for the evening. I was sick and unknowingly killing myself by improperly reducing the meds too quickly, the meds that reduce the swelling around my tumor. I wanted to get off these terrible meds that were bloating my belly and turning me into a moonfaced alien I didn't recognize in the mirror.

We stayed overnight with Connie, a long-time friend of Delynn's. Connie hosted a dinner for some of Delynn's friends (Shari, Lita, Evan, Tim, and Brian), whom I had not met. It was a fun night, but I felt terrible. The next day we visited Ken and Teresa, who presented us with a block with the quote from Jeremiah: 29:11: *I Know the Plans,* burned into the wood.

It finally dawned on me to up my dosage of Dex back to 4mg. Literally, within hours, I began feeling better. As all GBM cancer patients know, Dex is like wrestling with the devil. It keeps you alive, but it can kill you just as fast.

We didn't stay but three days in Nashville before jumping back in our white Hyundai and began the eight-hour journey to Roanoke.

~Chronicle 158

November 21, 2013, Cross County Trek to VB Roanoke, VA.

We stayed at another 100-year-old hotel, *the Roanoke*, a five-star Hotel. We had a glorious dinner, and the room mattresses were soft but firm. Tomorrow, we had only a five-hour drive to reach our new apartment in Virginia Beach. Now that I was stuffed to the gills with Dex, I was feeling a whole lot better.

We had some free time to relax in the hotel, so I used it to look through the postings on the Inspire Brain Tumor Board. I wondered, "Why aren't there any postings about the sex lives of GBM's? No one talks about it like it doesn't exist. My wife and I had a great sex life before GBM, but I lost any desire after diagnosis. For three long weeks, the tool was dead. A limp kite tail—it really did make me *feel* like I was dying.

A few years before, my wife and I discussed "what if" either one of us lost our ability or desire, how would we handle it? It made it easier to walk through the reality before us.

My sex drive did come around, but it took almost a month to kick back in. And when it did, I told Delynn, "You better take advantage of it while you still have a chance!" Take a personal note from me. If you can, keep your sex drive alive, your spouse needs it as much as you do. It is not a time for forced celibacy. For many of us, when we lose our vitality, we die.

The biggest threat to living longer is giving up. If there is no chance to survive, I'll stop trying. But if there is still a chance, bring on the sex. ~**Chronicle 161**~**Chronicle 162**

November 22, 2013, Cross County Trek to Virginia Beach, VA Arrival!

When we arrived in Virginia Beach at 1:00 p.m. the next day, to our surprise, the furniture had not yet arrived. We had no bed to sleep on, so my sister came to the rescue with a Queen-sized air mattress. They are never as comfortable as you would like, but we slept on it for two long nights, thankful to have arrived safely.

Delynn and I were tired, but we were home. Before I went to bed, I looked out the window and stared at King Neptune, our 34-foot Greek cast bronze icon who stood watch over the Virginia Beach sea. It was hard to believe I was here. Sand, old friends, church, and family. The only place I ever felt like home. ~**Chronicle 165**

November 25, 2013, Virginia Beach, VA

The furniture finally arrives. Only a few things were broken. Vacuum cleaner parts are missing. We'll have to buy a new one. Don't sweat the small stuff. Our new apartment is not Akio Gardens, but we are a block from the ocean. I am close to my family. My trees are safe. Now we just need to unpack. ~**Chronicle 167**

November 27, 2013, Virginia Beach, VA

Unpacking is done. Delynn had set up house as quickly as possible. She wanted us to "feel" settled in such a world of turmoil. Our apartment is only 1100 square feet. Humble again.

That's downsizing from our 4000 square foot home at Akio, in Washington. We have a nice 300 square-foot wooden deck overlooking the courtyard pool. At least my Bonsai have a nice view outside.

Even though we're "home," guilt pervaded my soul about leaving Benjamin and Angela with their mother in Washington. Did I make the right choice? Did I abandon my kids so I could die in VB? Why was I here?

Of course, there were other reasons: I felt like it was totally where I was supposed to be. There were possibilities for world-class GBM Treatment at Duke University, only a four-hour drive from VB. My family and church family near-by to help when times became hard. Still, I couldn't get the haunting doubts out of my mind...~*Chronicle 168*

November 28, 2013, Virginia Beach, VA

Thanksgiving Day. Delynn and I knocked on Mom's door and walked in. Delynn's son James had already arrived. Missing? Ben and Angela. My heart was sad. Even though Mom cooks the BEST Thanksgiving turkey, I wondered if Ben and Angela thought about the many years when "their Dad" always cooked Thanksgiving dinner. I'm sure their mother will fix a nice ham or goose, Canadian style.

Staring at the 25 lb browned Butterball turkey, I still pondered my decision to move to VB. It seemed logical. It seemed the path God had opened, and everything fell into place, and yet in all this terminal dying madness, I still felt empty without my children near my side.

Everything had happened so fast. Now we all are stuck with me dying three thousand miles away. I wonder if my kids and I will ever sit down for another Thanksgiving Dinner. There are many "is this the last time" thoughts that repeatedly happened over the next many months. I guess it's natural to think these thoughts when you are terminally ill. Cancer sucks. ~*Chronicle 172*

Before our arrival, Delynn had set up my first appointment for the VA – in Virginia. Though I was already under oncology care at the VA in Seattle, I had to go through a primary care physician to refer me to a new oncologist. We would need an appointment with the oncologist right away, before the next round of Temador Chemo that started December 1st. Delynn was prepared to get me the best treatment for Glioblastoma. Armed with a letter to the medical center prepared to explain why we needed therapy outside of the VA and the ramifications if we didn't get the proper treatment. She had already experienced the roadblock from the chemo department in Seattle. They refused to send me to experts in the field but had we stayed in Washington longer, the letter would have been submitted. Armed and ready, we entered the clinic and met with my new doctor, Dr. Vincent Lee. He reviewed my medical records and announced that he thought I should be referred to either Duke or John Hopkins. Delynn burst into tears. Our next step was to see the VA oncologist for an official referral.

We were sent to the oncologist the same day, at the Hampton Roads Medical Center, a place we would visit all too often. When we met with the oncologist, he was not friendly and seemed worn out, and had no sense of caring. He showed no initiative except he agreed Duke or John Hopkins should see me and since we had already talked with Dr. Freedman at Duke months prior. We chose Duke Medical Center.

It was quickly evident to Delynn that he was not like my primary doctor, who was a breath of fresh air. She had to be assertive. We still needed the Temador, but the doctor said there was no Temador at the facility, and it would be two weeks before they would have any. David needed some in two days!!

We asked whether we could buy it at our local pharmacy, which proved difficult and expensive. Delynn insisted he call the on-site pharmacy just to ask, even though the system said they had none. The pharmacy was located on the first floor of the same building. He reluctantly called.

They had precisely enough Temodar (chemo)—300mg a day for five days— for my December chemo treatments. Somebody up in Heaven is thinking about me. ~*Chronicle 173*

December 3rd. Delynn's newest grandbaby was born! He is a healthy baby boy. His name is Liam. It is also my sister Michelle's birthday. She turned 53. How's that for timing?

Note: After watching CNN's interview about Mary O'Neil's dramatic near-death experience yesterday, I wonder if there might be an opportunity to share my story? A little premature, don't you think, David? I can talk about my experience, but I don't have a book. The last three years of work had only given me *material; I had some chapters, many ideas but nothing cohesive. I have no credentials. I* have many Chronicle notes, writings and I still have nothing to give John Anthony West for review. I feel brain-fogged all the time from the chemo. How will I ever get the Chronicles done?

December 6, 2013, Trip to Atlantis, Bahamas

Delynn and I had purchased my sister's timeshare at Atlantis Bahamas at the beginning of 2013, before my diagnosis. We had no idea if we would get to use it. When my life was given an expiration date, I wanted to do a few things before I lost the ability to do so. My favorite thing to do was to snorkel and body surf in the tropics. Now that we lived on the East Coast, it was time to visit Atlantis in the Bahamas.

Our choice was limited to the first week of December. We wanted to bring the kids because they loved Atlantis, having been there two times before. But they were still in school. The timeshare had two bedrooms, so we invited our friends from Olympia to join us.

Sarah and Derrick's joy and youthful presence was just the medicine we needed.

We had gone to the pool/hot-tub the first evening we were there.

After a finger pruning two-hour soak in the hot tub, we got to know everyone—their jobs, where they lived, and why they were visiting such a lovely tropical place. Sometime after dusk, it came to my turn to talk about my life. I was still bald from radiation and never liked to mention my illness, but it came out anyway—the story about cancer and the Dead Saints Chronicles, which quickly became the hot topic of discussion.

As usual, no matter where we went, the subject of near-death research, writing, facing cancer, or death would come up in the conversation. People were open to sharing their stories, whether a visitation of a deceased loved one, a dream, or an encounter that was hard to explain, including their struggles of life, love, and loss.

We began to call our moments the "Hot Tub Conversations of the Afterlife."

A businessman named "Marc" shared his story when he was stabbed on a New York City street while on his way to a business meeting sometime during the 1980s. A man nearby who had just finished a drug deal ran over to help him after the assailant ran away. Blood was everywhere. The drug dealer flagged down a cab dragged him in, and together they rushed him to the hospital, an act that ultimately saved Marc's life.

He later discovered the dramatic event caused the drug dealer to give up drugs, and later, he became a paramedic. After Marc told the story, no one spoke for several minutes. Like my cancer, tragedy is sometimes part of God's plan. ~*Chronicle 176*

December 10, 2013, Atlantis, Bahamas

After several inner-tube float revolutions through river rapids, we got cold even though the water was 84 degrees.

We walked ½ mile to their main pool to eat lunch and lounge next to Atlantis' main pool that sits at the base of their notorious Mayan slide barrels through a shark aquarium. Sunning myself by the poolside, I watched the children playing in the pool, splashing and giggling, next to the "serious-faced adults" nearby.

It reminded me of Jesus saying, "Unless you are one of these children, you shall in no wise enter the kingdom of Heaven." ~**Chronicle 180**

December 23, 2013, Virginia Beach, VA

Ben and Angela are on a flight from Olympia to VB to be with me for Christmas, but their flight was delayed overnight. I knew the kids were experienced travelers, but no parent likes their kids stuck at the airport by themselves. They arrive safely but tired. ~**Chronicle 193**

Personal thought: Salvation is not a "get out of jail free card," allowing us to do anything we want. Jesus still forgives our sins and wipes our slate clean, separating our sins, "As far apart as the East is from the West." But remember, we still live in a cause/effect universe. Those laws still apply. ~**Chronicle 195**

December 25, Virginia Beach, VA

Delynn jammed what used to be 4000 square feet of Christmas decorations into our small apartment, 1100 square foot apartment.

It looked like a Christmas store! Opening presents and Christmas ham with the family and the kids. Thank you, Lord, for all blessings you have bestowed upon us. We are not perfect, but we love one another. ~**Chronicle 197**

December 27 MRI at the Hampton, VA medical Center. 45 minutes of boredom. I hope the MRI is clear. We have to send a copy of the MRI disk to Duke University for the neuro-oncologist to review. ~**Chronicle 198**

December 28, 2013, Virginia Beach, VA

The kids fly back to the West Coast but will meet their mother along the way in Cabo, Mexico, for a warm vacation on their way home to Olympia, Washington. Strangely, their flight got delayed overnight again, but they arrived safe...~**Chronicle 202**

January 1, 2014, Virginia Beach, VA

I survived to see another New Year's celebration. Will I reach 2015? New Year's brunch at Bruce and Marty's home. Met the local Seer, Joy Talley. Joy Talley's story is written in the chapter, Near-Death Lightening, a description of an encounter with Jesus. ~**Chronicle 204**

I delivered the sermon, 'A Mission from God,' the first I had given since before Paul Solomon died. Standing at the podium with my Ministers robe and stole set in motion a new life I could never have imagined. I finished the sermon with a new relationship with Christ. Thank you, Lord, for believing in me.

Part II

Training Wires

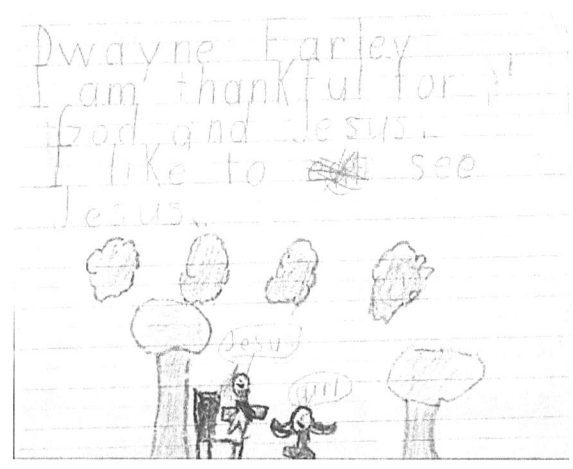

We were not religious. I don't remember the words "God" or "Jesus" in any conversation, except during the Christmas season. Then it was Santa Claus we celebrated, and presents, and decorating the Christmas tree. Yet, years later, in my baby book, mom rediscovered a crayon picture I'd drawn at age seven. It was of Jesus holding a girl's hand under a tree.

― 7 ―

The Foundation Wires

California Beginnings

I was born in Greenbrae hospital, San Rafael, California, on January 23, 1959, a city to the north of San Francisco at the base of 4000-foot Mount Tamalpais. I was a normal healthy baby, but tongue-tied at birth, a defect easily remedied by the obstetrician's scissors' snip.

Early life was a whirlwind. We had moved multiple times, crisscrossing the country. Most of our time was spent in California, where my mother's family was. My dad was first in the Air Force; then, after many attempts to find gainful employment, he joined the Navy.

I have brief memories when attending 1st & 2nd grade in Coronada, California, near the Mexican border. I remember almost nothing about it except standing and reciting the Pledge of Allegiance and doing "tuck and cover" drills if we were the target of a Russian nuclear attack.

I spent a lot of time in the woods, getting to know the snakes, frogs, tadpoles, and forest life. Living in the solitude of the forest helped mold me. I shied away from strangers and often wandered alone among the trees bordering our backyard, accompanied only by our German shepherd, foraging for wild huckleberries. No smartphones, texting, or much TV in those days. Saturday morning cartoons, *Johnny Quest*, and waiting a year for the *Wizard of Oz* or *Rudolph the Red Nose Reindeer* to air again-- if we could get the rabbit ears and tin foil to work or keep the lights glowing in the TV's vacuum tubes.

First Intimations, Early Glimpses

We were not religious.

I don't remember the words "God" or "Jesus" ever in any conversation, except at Christmas, and even then it was about Santa Claus we celebrated, presents, decorating the Christmas tree.

Yet, years later, in my baby book, mom rediscovered a crayon picture I'd drawn aged seven of Jesus holding a girl's hand under a tree. It was cute but very odd. Santa Claus would have been more appropriate.

It must have been when I was six or seven, during the Christmas season, that I tried to fix a broken Christmas light with a screwdriver, which promptly blew up and melted the tip. Back then, Christmas lights were big bulbs with 120 volts of hot electricity flowing through them. I was alone, and it was only by the "grace of God" that I was not electrocuted. It was not a classic NDE, a dramatic departure from this planet, and subsequent miraculous return. But I could easily have been killed.

In 1967, at eight, I realized I felt and acted differently from the other kids. I was a quick study in school with a voracious appetite for reading, mostly science fiction about space travel and anything astronomy. I was a dreamer, but yet a scientist at heart, which would subsequently drive my lifelong passion for research.

I was 11, in late December 1970, when the Navy relocated us to Norfolk, Virginia. It was a big move; I remember being so excited. It was like moving to another planet. We arrived in late December in an ice storm and quickly bought a small two-story house in Virginia Beach for $17,000.

When I look back on my early years, I think, when Dad came home from his long Navy tours overseas, he took his frustrations out on me. With Dad, I felt I could never do anything right. Mom always seemed to be there to protect me from him and fixed dinner every night. I was afraid of him. That's what I remember.

The relationship between mom and dad was always rocky, with most arguments revolving around money or its lack. I had no clue about what was going on. But in the spring of 1971, family life seemed to improve. We began attending the United Church of Christ pastored by Tracy Floyd. I think the stresses of their married life drove them to find a church where God could help them work out their relationship. It was a small, family-oriented protestant church with a strong Christ-centered message. I know Mom and Dad found God there because Dad went through a very emotional catharsis, remorse about things he had done earlier in his life. I remember lots of crying and the church congregation physically hugging him and forgiving him, with lots of prayer and drama.

I looked forward to church services every Sunday. It wasn't long before pastor Tracy noticed I had a love for scripture and God, and it was during those years that I began to develop a deep love and trust in Him.

Astronaut Aspirations

My family acknowledged me as a scientist, astronomer, and dreamer. I intended to become the first man to Mars. In 1974, when I turned 15, I began grinding my own mirror for an eight-inch 64" focal length reflector telescope—a project that still sits in a dusty box in my closet. I was a gung-ho Galilean scientist. I hung small, painted planets from my ceiling.

I memorized everything about the solar system, the number of moons revolving around the planets, their revolution rate, mass, gravity, and distance from the Sun. No one told me to do it, nor did anyone help me. I just loved science.

USAF

My goal back then was to become an astronaut. My family had no money. Even though I was an honor graduate with a 3.4-grade point average, I was on my own. I received no advice about scholarships, and it didn't occur to me to ask. For me, it was Air Force Academy or bust. I intended to become a Test Pilot, and then eventually an astronaut. I went through the Air Force Academy application process, but my SAT scores weren't good enough. My application was rejected. I was crushed.

I had no plan "B" for college. I just didn't have the money to pay for tuition. My future, my dreams, and my goals were suddenly dashed to pieces. It felt like the scientist in me died that day. So what does a dead scientist do?

As a Navy vet, my dad suggested enlisting in the US Air Force since that would make me eligible for matching education funds. It seemed like my only option. So, I took the Air Force entrance test, scored in the top 1%, and signed up under the "Veterans Delayed Enlistment Program" while still in my senior year in high school, intending to enter active service after graduating September 1977.

After Basic Training at Lackland AFB, in Texas, I had to choose the job I would perform in my Air Force career. Since neither becoming an astronaut or scientist were options for an enlisted man in the Air Force, I chose electronics, something I was at least familiar with; I had previously taken three years of electronics in high school.

My commanding officer, however, had other ideas for me. My high test scores qualified me for another career in the Air Force I never knew existed – nor was it customarily made available to an 18-year-old.

"Airman!" I stood at attention. "Yes, sir!"

"Do you want to fly?"

What? "Would you be interested in flying?" I couldn't believe what I was hearing.

"Yes, sir!"

"We are offering you a position as a B-52 gunner. You will be an enlisted member of the six-man flight crew. You will receive flight pay and additional off-base benefits. What say you?" I had always wanted to be an astronaut and become a Test Pilot. I guess this was God's way of getting me as close to my life goals as I could imagine. Of course, I said, "Yes. Sign me up." I had no idea what I would face.

Conscientious Objector

B-52 gunners are required to receive a Top Secret clearance, which I subsequently accepted. I later discovered Secret Service agents visited my neighborhood in Virginia Beach and interviewed friends and family as they researched my background. That was scary. It was nothing serious to uncover about my life other than typical high school pranks that I am not proud of, but I guess I was clean enough.

I trained in B-52 gunner's school at Castle AFB near Merced, California, and graduated top of my class. My job entailed defending the Aircraft from MIGs trying to shoot us down as we entered Russia, drop Nuclear Weapons on Russian cities, finish what the Intercontinental nukes had missed some thirteen hours earlier, a WW III scenario. It was what I trained for, and it was the only thing we planned for. I was only 18, yet I was responsible for monthly flight plans and briefings attended by generals regularly.

We were on "alert" seven days a week, and when the claxons went off, we never knew if it was a drill or if WWIII was starting. In theory, we had just minutes to get off the ground before Russian submarine nukes hit our base. I sat next to the Electronics Warfare officer, who received the "authentication" codes from SAC "Strategic Air Command" for a "fly or no-fly" decision.

Of course, the codes never authorized us to take off to drop our nukes, and we always assumed it was a drill, but...you never knew for sure.

I remember inspecting the B-52's, touching their nuclear weapons, and wondering, "Wow, this is really against everything I ever believed in. - What am I doing here? Yes. I was flying, but to be a part of killing millions of people was a nagging question that became a moral and spiritual nightmare for me.

Dark Night of the Soul

By September 1979, after 18 months of military service in the USAF, I faced a moral dilemma I could not resolve; how can I be a spiritual person and still be a part of a military operation that potentially could kill millions of people? My job in the Air Force had been a B-52 gunner, where I had faced World War III scenarios regularly. After months of intense emotional conflict, I filed for Conscientious Objector status with my flight crew's agreement.

It was not a light or easy decision. I had been at the top of my B-52 1977 Gunner class with options to enter the US Air Force Academy. I had intended to become an astronaut since I was seven. Joining the Air Force Academy was an essential step towards fulfilling that dream. But when I was handed my DD-Form 214 granting my honorable discharge, I knew my career as a "spaceman" was over.

I hung up my flight suit and departed Griffiths Air Force Base in March. The long 12-hour drive from Rome, New York to Virginia Beach, Virginia, still left me little time to think about my future career.

For the first time in my life, I felt rudderless. I had no clue what I was going to do with my life. I had always steered in the direction of the stars; now, I was earthbound.

I toyed with going to college, but there was no money for tuition. I don't know if it was depression or if I just gave up. To this day, I am not sure why I did not pursue a scholarship. My younger sister Terri did and landed one that paid for four years of college.

I think, in the end, I was angry at God that my life's dream to be an astronaut was at an end. It is not like me to give up so quickly, but for some reason, I did. In an attempt to drown in my sorrows, I drove to a nearby 7-11 and bought a couple of six-packs, drove into the middle of my mother's front lawn, got drunk, and began yelling at God.

The yelling became screaming at the top of my lungs, "God, what do you want me to do with my life?"

Tears streaming down my face, the supplication intensified. "I demand that you tell me what I am going to do with my life!" Years of failed life purpose poured out of me. What was I going to do? I cried out from the depths of my soul. I reached down so deep with so much emotion, hoping against all hope that my anger would somehow get His attention.

It was the dark night of my soul. It was a plea for help, a plea for answers, and a plea for direction sent at light-speed throughout the universe.

The date was April 15, 1979. I was 20. You may have noticed; I still held my birth name, Dwayne M. Earley. Though I did not realize it consciously, God's training wires were tightening around my soul, creating the "Nebari" —the roots that became the foundation of my journey, which would become an integral part of *The Dead Saints Chronicles*.

~First, we must recognize God speaking to us in the outer, physical world. When we begin to see his Light in the flower, the Bonsai, and trees, and the daily breadcrumbs, God sets before us, in the chance meeting with people, and the words they speak, we will begin to open the veil to the inner life of Christ's Light within. Since the light within us is Love, it can only transform our lives. How do we know the voice of God when we have so many screaming voices in our heads? If we pay attention to the quiet miracles happening around us every day— God's trumpets – they are still and small – but it is God speaking to us. To know Him ever so closely requires a daily walk with Him. ~**Chronicle 245**

8

The Founders

Teachers

May 30, 1979

New Market, Virginia

When you are told you have a terminal illness, past events come under close scrutiny least they did in my case, and I do not think I am an exception. As we look back and review our lives, we may wonder how our bonsai was pruned and styled by significant events, parents, friends, tragedy, and even luck.

Important training wires of my soul were molded and shaped by the nearly 13 years spent with Paul Solomon—the Rice Paper Teacher I introduced to you in Book I. There is much more to tell. I did not have space to write about the first book, so this chapter is the "rest of our story."

In late May 1979, two months after my honorable discharge as a Conscientious Objector, browsing in at the ARE (Association for Research and Enlightenment) bookstore, I stumbled upon a little booklet, *Ether Technology"* by Rho Sigma (obviously a pen name). It was a dissertation on faster-than-light travel and New Science technologies. I was interested in UFOs at this time in my life, and I picked up the book. Poring through, I came across a curious excerpt at near the end of the book quoted from *The Paul Solomon Tapes*, where the author Rho Sigma writes, "A fairly new psychic with enormous potential, Paul Solomon, called the "Second Edgar Cayce" by some, and living now in Virginia Beach, like Edgar Cayce before him, confirms these statements [about the discovery of a new understanding of

Physics, and how we could learn to float heavy objects through the air, much like heavy objects floating in water]." [6]

What floored me: Paul Solomon was called the "Second Edgar Cayce" and lived in Virginia Beach. I had studied Edgar Cayce's readings for many years, but Cayce was dead. Paul Solomon was alive and living in Virginia Beach, and at first glance appeared to be able to do the same things for which Edgar Cayce was famous.

I asked the bookstore clerk if she knew Paul Solomon. She said he was a local Christian Minister who pastored the Fellowship of the Inner Light, a small research study center on 37th Street,[7] literally just a mile from where I was standing. It only took minutes to get there.

Paul Solomon wasn't there. He lived in New Market, a few hundred miles to the West, in the Shenandoah Valley. – No matter. The group at the Center invited me in, and within days, I was listening to years of cassette tapes filled with Paul's lectures and readings.

Paul, born William Dove, and a fourth-generation Southern Baptist Ministers, was from the Bible Belt's buckle, where the ministry is the assumed career. Paul's great-grandfather was one of the old "circuit-rider" preachers during the expansion of the West. Paul described him as "a preacher with a Bible in one hand, Colt Peacemaker in the other, for snakes...of all kinds."[8]

Growing up, he watched his parents seek guidance daily and noted they based decisions on the silent replies they received. God was accessible; the Holy Spirit was an active participant in their everyday lives.

---

[6] Rho Sigma, *Ether-Technology: a rational approach to gravity-control*, published by Rho Sigma, 1986, p. 104.
[7] The Fellowship later relocated to 620 14th Street, Virginia Beach
[8] Description of Paul's great-grandfather excerpted from: Michael McCarthy 2012. *On Death and Living: Memoir of a Soul*. Virginia Beach, VA: Paul Solomon Institute Publications. p. 154.

As a child, being exposed to fundamentalist Christian beliefs, he was taught and believed God was always available for guidance and took comfort in that belief.

But for the young Paul Solomon, there was a hitch, a genuine dilemma. He exhibited uncommon abilities that did not jibe with the Baptist life. From an early age, he saw colors around people. He called them "good lights" and "bad lights," depending on how he perceived the individual. He would point at someone and sound the alarm, "He's bad!" His embarrassed parents would scold him for being rude. Eventually, he learned to keep what he saw to himself. He knew what people were thinking and learned early that most people say the opposite. He also knew about events beforehand; he could predict the future, which frustrated and undermined his attempt to be "like everyone else." While these "gifts of knowledge," these psychic experiences, came naturally to Paul, they were not "normal."

At 14, he was ordained. He began his pastoral tasks by ministering to the incarcerated and their families as the youngest Baptist Minister in the Arkansas Prison system. Soon after high school, Paul enlisted in the Army, married, and had a daughter. After the Army, he enrolled in a Baptist Seminary. During this period, Paul preached in a Spanish speaking Mexican Baptist church in the Panhandle of Texas. He was well on this way to a successful career when his wife filed for divorce, leaving him for another man. Back in 1967, there was no such thing as a divorced Southern Baptist Minister. So in one day, he lost his family and his career.

The traumatic experience left him very, very angry at God. He had given over his entire life to serving the Lord, and he felt God had pulled the rug out from under him. And he rebelled; first smoking, then drinking. Southern Baptists don't even use wine for communion. It was an entirely new experience.

He spent the next five years working, partying, trying not to think about God, and surrounding himself with people who were doing the same.

One day, watching his pet hamsters running endlessly on their treadmill, the lesson struck home: "That's me." he thought. "I am running as hard as I can just to keep myself from thinking about my life." With that sudden realization and little further ado, he kicked out the roommates he'd been partying with and went into seclusion. He closed the blinds, locked his door, and stopped answering the phone.

He had an evening job as a nightclub manager and still reported to work, but his life had gone from frenetic activity to avoiding everybody. Days were spent in the dark in his apartment, and nights locked in his night club office. For about thirty days, the night club ran itself, which the waitresses loved.

He began to worry about his sanity. Maybe someone could tell him "he was alright" and help him out of unrelenting depression. At his Seminary, he had majored in psychology, but he did not think a doctor could give him useful answers. He didn't want to talk to a Minister because he knew what they would say. Then he remembered his work in the Army at the Brooke Army Medical Center. Under doctors' supervision, he had been part of a pilot program that used hypnosis in battlefield situations when pain killers were not available. He had also witnessed hypnosis help soldiers through a variety of personal problems, including depression. And given the success of that program, he thought that a good hypnotherapist would help him. He found a hypnosis clinic in the yellow pages, called and made an appointment. The therapist seemed confident that Paul's problem was a deep-seated guilt complex by his strict religious upbringing and was sure that successful treatment was possible. However, when Paul was told the exorbitant price of the twice-weekly sessions, he left feeling more miserable than ever. Even when he actively sought help, it remained out of reach. His life was at a crisis point.

Hypnosis Experiment Triggers a Near-Death Experience

Paul went to work one night angry and bitter, but at least he had finally talked about his problem. He revealed his predicament to Harry Snipes, a regular at the nightclub. "How in the world I supposed to afford hypnosis at those prices?" he complained.

"I hypnotized someone once," Harry offered, his voice trailing off as Paul ranted on about the unfairness of life. Incredulous, Paul stared at him.

"You hypnotized someone once?" he echoed.

There was dubious confidence in Harry's expression, and Paul supposed "once" could happen again. "Let's go, then!" And off they went to Paul's apartment where he laid down, closed his eyes, and submitted, with no apprehension, to Harry's unprofessional instructions. Paul's last conscious thought was, "This'll never work. This guy has no idea what he's doing. If anything happens, it'll be because he bored me to sleep."

The night was February 14, 1972. In response to Harry's bland attempts at hypnotism, Paul appeared to fall asleep. Without warning, his body jerked erect as if his soul had been shot from a cannon out of his body. He began speaking in an intense, authoritative voice, apparently unconscious on the couch. Paul awoke from the hypnosis session, doubled up with pain from cramps in his stomach, and Harry jumping up and down with excitement insisting they had talked to "spirits."

His only recollection of the hypnosis session upon awaking was a dream, which would later be recognized as some of the "classic" core death elements of the near-death experience:

I am approaching the entrance to a tunnel. It is similar to the mouth of a cornucopia because it seems to spiral inward and upward. I can see two figures at the opening. They seem to be waiting for me. One is Merle, who was my girlfriend in high school until she died in our senior year. The other is my young friend, Jaida, who remained my secret companion for years following his death when we were seven. They each take me by the hand and lead me through the tunnel. We come out the other side onto a grassy hill. As we begin to climb, I see that we are approaching a temple at the top of the hill.... The two figures are waiting to take me through the tunnel. As I come out the other side, I find myself in a meadow of wildflowers where a soft breeze blows, and I can hear the sound of a brook. Ahead of me is a mountain. As I climb, I pass through seven terraced gardens of glorious color. At the top, I enter a temple. The air is rich with music, though I see no one. I see rows and rows of books with names on the bindings. I am in an enormous library.[9]

As Paul recovered from the violent post-session stomach cramps, Harry recalled all he could hear was "THE VOICE" —which to Paul, sounded too "religious" to be true.

He said, "Harry, what do you expect to get when you hypnotize an ex-Southern Baptist Preacher?" He didn't want to hear more and told Harry to leave. But Harry returned the next day, insisting they try the hypnosis experiment again. He pushed Paul for about a week until Harry made a remark that intrigued him.

He said, "Paul, I know that wasn't you because you're not that smart."

The next time Harry brought a tape recorder, and together they formulated a test question; a question that neither knew the answer to but that was provable. Paul wanted to make sure that the answer was not coming from his subconscious mind.

[9] Paul Solomon Reading excerpt, February 21, 1972.

Paul's great grandfather had been murdered before Paul was born and died without disclosing the whereabouts of a large sum of money he had been saving but hiding. In spite of a thorough search, the family had never found the money.

The question: "Where was Great Grandfather's money?"

They set up another hypnosis session to clarify "who" was talking, and this time recorded it. Again, the authoritative, booming voice spoke:

You have not attained sufficient growth or spiritual awareness to understand these records...That which you perform is a foolish experiment, for you attempt to harness powers you do not understand and to contact sources, records, and intelligences' you are not familiar with, how will you try the spirits should you attain that you seek? Would you recognize Him, whom you do not know, have not been familiar with?[10]

During hypnosis, the "conductor" asked Paul, "Who is speaking?" Paul stated emphatically:

This is not a spirit. It is not some other personality. You are talking with the Source of his Mind, which gave birth to his mind. It pre-existed his physical body and created his physical body.[11]

Harry asked the voice what they should do to prepare spiritually for further hypnosis sessions.

They were given a list of instructions, including a specific diet, exercise, prayer, meditation, and a recommendation to read the Sacred Scriptures in the Bible and study the *Search for God* books from the A.R.E. Harry asked, "What's the ARE?" The voice explained Edgar Cayce's organization, the Association for Research and Enlightenment in Virginia Beach, Virginia.

---

[10] Paul Solomon Reading Excerpt, February 21, 1972.
[11] Ibid.

This time when Paul awoke, he was able to listen to the voice on tape. He heard a strong, more authoritative version of his own voice, providing detailed information on several subjects, including a thorough description of his great grandfather's death and the whereabouts of the hidden money: in the chimney of the old family home. *(The money was later retrieved by Reverend Dove, Paul's father. Attempts to identify the amount of Grampa's stash were unsuccessful, primarily because he kept it a private family matter).*

The voice also explained the stomach cramps Paul experienced upon returning to ordinary consciousness:

Your consciousness is disengaging itself from the physical body. When the physical body feels the consciousness leaving, it associates that with death and will do anything in its power to hold consciousness in the body. And for that reason, those muscles are cramping in an attempt to sustain life.[12]

After the session, as a kind of finale, the voice described a man who addressed a comment to Reverend Dove—Paul's father; *"You will know who this is and you'll remember our agreement, and that this is the conclusion of our agreement."* Paul realized he had never encountered anything like this during his Southern Baptist Ministry. He knew this wasn't just religion emanating from his own subconscious. He was both excited and disturbed by it.

But he needed to know: Was this of God?

So with the cassette tape in hand, he went to South Carolina to consult the man whom he most trusted to know the answer, the Southern Baptist Preacher who would know: his father, the Reverend Dove.

---

[12] Ibid.

After playing the tape, he asked his father, "So, is it of God, or is it of the Devil?" Looking him straight in the eye, his father didn't hesitate and said, "*It's of God.*"

Paul, playing Devil's advocate, asked, "Dad, how can you say that? Southern Baptists don't believe in this stuff."

The Reverend replied, "There are two reasons I know it's of God. You know, this is not the first time in history that something like this has occurred. The prophet Daniel found himself in a situation where his life depended on receiving word from God regarding the interpretation of King Nebuchadnezzar's disturbing dream— information that was not available to his conscious mind. Under threat of death, he went into a room with his three friends, and according to the Bible story, he 'prayed all night.' I believe after their prayers, Daniel laid down and went to sleep, and he awoke in the morning with the dream's true meaning, which he passed on to the king, saving their lives. It seems to me that Daniel did something like what you just did."

His father continued, "And the second reason is this: ever since you left the ministry five years ago, your mother and I have prayed every day for God to find a way to bring you back to a right relationship with Him. I knew it had to be something dramatic. I know it's of God because, "I asked God for bread, and I know God did not give us a scorpion or a stone."[13]

Reverend Dove advised Paul to go back to Atlanta and carefully pursue his ministry. He expressed his belief that every minister when he stands before a congregation, represents himself as communicating with God and should have that ability.

---

[13]Matt 7: 9-10. "Or what man is there of you, whom if his son ask bread, will he give him a stone? Or if he asks for a fish, will he give him a serpent?"

Finally, he shared with Paul the meaning of the little reference at the end of the tape. Twenty-five years earlier, Reverend Dove discussed with a friend about whether or not there was awareness after death. His father's response at the time was that he didn't know, but they both were intrigued by the possibility of life after death. The two of them agreed that whichever one passed on first, if possible, they would attempt to make contact and communicate. So the message on the tape was the completion of their agreement made over two decades before.

The encounter with "the Source," as he would later call it, was for Paul Solomon, a life-transforming experience. He found that what had begun by accident, he could later duplicate at will. Paul's "Source reading" trance state was verified at the J.B. Rhine Institute for Parapsychological Studies at Duke University in 1972. Researchers found that Paul could enter the unconscious Delta Brain Wavefield (0.5 to 4 cycles per second) and still speak, astounding the doctors monitoring him.

His "Source readings" and later his lectures and classes became the catalyst for a worldwide ministry. At the time, I had no clue Paul's own NDE and life's work would become a basis for my studies and writing thirty years later in the Dead Saints Chronicles' writing. I had cried out with all my heart to God just a week before pleading with God for help. I, too, believed I would be given bread instead of a stone—because I asked. However, at the time, it never occurred to me that God had answered my "What-do-you-want-me-to-do-with-my-life?" ravings from just a week earlier. Events were just "passing by" at life speed. I was only conscious of those things right in front of me.

Should I be Ordained?

Paul had developed a Seminary where ministers were ordained. God was a central part of my life. I'd just been honorably discharged from the Air Force as a conscientious objector for my beliefs. I chewed long and hard upon the idea. It was not long before the question turned into a real possibility. "Should I be? Could I be ordained?"

It was not an alien notion. Back in '75, Pastor Tracy suggested I might want to become a minister. It was an attractive idea, but at that time, I still had astronaut aspirations. I loved God, but I was not ready to commit to a life of service as a man of the cloth.

The Fellowship had organized a major conference in late August, *The Spirit of Friendship*, in the Shenandoah Valley. It was one of the largest inter-faith and metaphysical conferences ever assembled, attracting well-known teachers, including Elisabeth Kübler-Ross, Donald Keys, Sir George Travelyan, Buckminster Fuller, Swami Kriyandanda, Alan Chadwick, and hundreds of laypeople from around the world. I felt it was imperative for my future to attend the conference. It was not just a matter of getting there. I owned a car. But in such a throng of people, I was no one of importance. Who would pay attention to me or care about my needs or my experiences?

A few weeks before, I'd had a vivid dream about visiting a large auditorium with my mother to hear Paul deliver a speech. An angel was standing on the stage next to him, but before the talk could begin, the angel walked down the aisle, stepped into the row in which we were seated, and proceeded to ask my mother for "permission" for me to leave her so I could be Paul's "student." She agreed because I woke up from the dream "knowing" that Paul would be my teacher.

I quickly formed a plan. I wrote a sincere, long, soppy letter addressed to Paul, requesting ordination, and dropped it in the mail, expecting it to arrive just before the Conference.

Three days later, I drove up to New Market, hoping the letter would be placed in Paul's hands and that he would read it.

I was right.

I waited all afternoon by the white colonial mansion's swimming pool, the 1600 acre headquarters of the Fellowship's Carmel-in-the-Valley garden, and Seminary School. Late in the day, Paul Solomon's assistant tracked me down.

He grinned at me. "You must be Dwayne. Yes. Paul read your letter. Follow me." Stephan marched me into the house into a vast, ornate 1920's windowed room with high ceilings, where Paul sat behind a desk, holding my letter. My letter included a sloppy, hand-written interpretation of *the Book of Revelation* I had composed during my service in the Air Force. It was a line by line, chapter by chapter, interpretation of the Book of Revelation based on Readings given by Edgar Cayce. Staring at my paper, Paul said, "So you are a Revelation scholar?"

I shrugged my shoulders. "It's just something I felt compelled to write."

He was quiet for a few moments and then said, "To be recognized as a teacher, the first thing you need to do is write a book to establish your credibility."

Six months after my honorable discharge from the USAF as a conscientious Objector, writing a book was the last thing I ever imagined I could do. Even though I loved writing, I considered my amateur skills incapable of such a task. A bit intimidated by Paul, I just nodded in agreement. At 20-years-old, it seemed a daunting order, but the vision of it stuck like glue in my mind.

Paul continued, "The Fellowship of the Inner Light has a two-year Gospel Ministry Ordination program." I will recommend to the Pastoral Council that your letter serves as your initial application to Seminary. When do you want to start?"

"I have no tuition money."

"You can work in exchange for tuition."

The boat anchor of reality fell with a thud to the floor. I was committing in that very moment to becoming a man of the cloth. The river of the universe was opening up, and I was jumping on God's giant yellow leaf and beginning a journey towards an unknown yet exciting destination.

"I need to sell my car...but I should be able to back up here within two weeks."

And with that, the meeting was over. My "Letter to Paul" mission accomplished, I drove back home to Virginia Beach. The meeting was magical. As planned, I made it back to the Shenandoah Valley. I didn't stay at the large Carmel-in-the-Valley, but instead, resided a few miles up the road at the Seminary School called Hearthfire Lodge.

After my arrival in mid-September, my life became a blur. My scribbled Book of Revelation notes went into a box, which sadly was lost, perhaps for good reason. In its place, I wrote a complete thesis 35 years later, which is included in Book III, the Armageddon Stones.

By late October, I was traveling with Paul Solomon, in Australia, as his assistant. Seminary classes had begun.

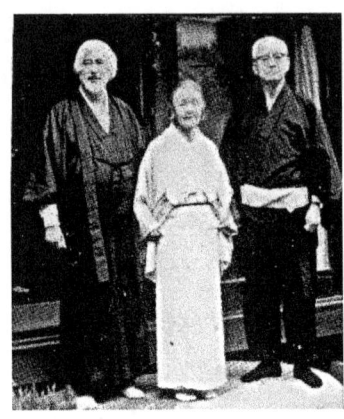

~I gave a sermon at the Fellowship, "Training Wires of the Soul." I wore the black 100-year-old silk Shinto robe given to Paul Solomon by Mr. Watanabe during our visit to Japan in 1988. Pictured to the left, Paul is wearing Mr. Watanabe's Robe. After Paul Solomon died in 1994, Sharon Solomon gave the Shinto Robe to me. I brought my Western Juniper bonsai to the service and set it on a small stand on the right side of the altar, and a picture of Jesus on the left side of the altar. Dick Dingus sent me a photo of the communion circle after the service. He pointed out in the photo a curious white orb floating six inches over my head. Maybe it was an angel? ~**Chronicle 267 (March 7, 2014)**

── 9 ──

The Form

Tao Wires

I had a life-altering encounter with a homeless bag lady on the streets of New York City. The electric experience brought me to my knees. It didn't happen because I believed she was Jesus Christ. It just happened. Who would expect a bag lady to be Jesus? I only smiled at her, and she responded with a smile and Holy Spirit smack in the heart!

But New York City had more training wires to apply to my bonsai I want to share with you.

In September 1980, Paul Solomon recommended that I and another student from Hearthfire, Andrew (nicknamed Billy), to a two-year study in New York City. Our planned curriculum consisted of journalism, business, typing, memory enhancement, speed reading, and T'ai Chi with Chinese Master Da Liu.

I was packing my bags to leave for NYC when Paul Solomon came upstairs and handed me $900. It bought me a train ticket NYC, rent a for a roach-infested apartment, buy a ten-speed bike, food, and school books, and time to track down a Tai Chi Master.

He also gave me three pages of brown parchment rolled like an ancient scroll. He said, "During your studies, read this scroll three times every day for forty days and forty nights. Make it part of your daily life. By the time your forty days are finished, you will have memorized the entire scroll word for word. Continue reciting it for as long as you stay in New York."

The scroll didn't look ancient; in fact, it looked brand new. It was called The Garden Scroll. I asked Paul, "When did you write this?"

He smiled, "When you became my student."

Paul stared at me, and in one of those rare moments, he began to talk about all of the wise "stuff" everyone else always seemed to get the opportunity to listen to because I had been busy as his assistant.

"The purpose of this scroll, *Dweeper* (my given nickname from Paul), is to convey the same message passed down by the Apostle Paul when he exhorted us to, 'not be conformed to this world, but transformed by the renewing of our minds.' You see, great men of history have often written about their struggle to reach transformation after their initial "God Experience." Paul wrote years after his encounter with the Christ on the road to Damascus, "The good that I would, I do not, and that I would not, I do."

St. Paul describes the transformation process by saying it was a daily path, "I am crucified with Christ; nevertheless I (the Father in me) live, yet not I (the personality) but Christ (Son of God) lives in me." Paul Solomon reminded me of St. Paul's exhortation to "die daily" to the competing thoughts of the lower mind, which distracts us from donning the divine mind of Christ.

Paul said, "That's the purpose of the Garden Scroll. By reading it three times a day, twice silently, once a loud in the evening, you will plant new seed thoughts into the garden of your heart and mind, so you can begin thinking, not with your lower mind, but with your higher mind, the mind of Christ. But you must first develop a point of reference for what that greater mind is like. You must begin to communicate with the Mind of Christ and build familiarity with how

He thinks. You must begin to call on this greater mind to make decisions. Eventually, you will start to depend more and more on that mind for your thought processes until the greater portion of your thinking originates there. The point of enlightenment comes when the lesser mind dies, and the greater mind of Christ becomes your Source of thought."

"Dweeper" transformation is a life-long task. Don't be hard on yourself. In Japan, some bonsai are trained over hundreds of years. Be patient."

And with that, Paul hugged me and said goodbye.

"I promise I will read the scroll every day."

"Make sure Billy recites the scroll."

"I will."

My mind was reeling. "Paul, thank you. I will do my best."

He smiled as I carefully packed the document into my already stuffed luggage and jumped into an old Subaru wagon, where a good friend, another student at Hearth fire, was waiting to drive me to Washington D.C. to make the connecting train. When I got on the train, the first thing I did was pull out the Garden Scroll. I arrived in NYC with my two eighty-pound bags. Only handles in those archaic pre-roller days. I had to stop every hundred feet to rest but managed to make way to my destination.

Billy and I had a job pre-arranged, with Dr. Warren M. Levin, Medical Director of the World Health Medical Group, a long-time acquaintance of Paul Solomon. Dr. Levin offered us additional work as "houseboys," cleaning and cooking, and ironing clothes— something I became very, very good at, a skill my wife appreciates even today.

However, we still needed a place to live. Together, with only nine hundred dollars between us in cash, we could not be choosy and considered ourselves "lucky" to find an old hotel converted to apartments on 110th and Broadway, two tiny bedrooms, and a grubby, roach-infested kitchen at $495 a month. That was the best we could afford.

We didn't have much: a few pots, pans, clothes, and some food. The rent included fresh sheets and towels once a week. Billy and I were a tag team. He would work six months while I went to school, and then we would switch, and he would study.

I took business typing and stenography classes at Berkley-Claremont business school. I was the only male among fifty female students, which was needless to say, a distraction, considerably aggravated when I fell in love with one of them. I enrolled in several individual night courses: journalism, Harry Loraine memory, and speed reading training, and time management among them. At the time, I had no idea how important these skills would become when I turned to research, writing, and eventually building the business that changed my life.

As promised, we read the Garden Scroll three times a day. What was funny was the "reading aloud" part, when I sometimes stuck my head out the window and shouted it out loud into the night air.

Tai Chi Master

While Paul had set out the basic daily routine, which included reading the Garden Scroll three times a day, it turned out that our trip's primary purpose was to become T'ai Chi students of Da Liu, the famous master. The latter brought the ancient martial art to America.

But we didn't know where he lived, other than that it was in upper Manhattan.

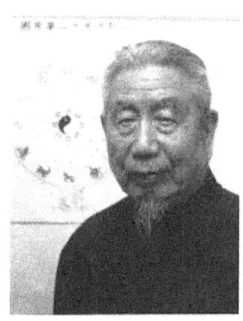
Of course, there was no internet back then. I didn't even think to look in the phone book. I asked around at some of the nearby fruit and vegetable shops. Had anyone heard of a Chinese Da Liu and his T'ai Chi classes? Someone suggested checking out Columbia University up on 120th street. "It's a big place to look around!" But I finally found a clerk in the administrative office who knew the name but thought he taught at the Cathedral of St. John the Divine down on 110th and Amsterdam.

Back I hiked. I asked the girl who took money for the Cathedral Tours if she knew where the Tai Chi classes were taught. She wasn't sure but directed me to the administrative office, where, at last, an elderly lady had an answer.

"Oh, well, right here," she said.

I got the class schedule and showed up with Billy for our first class a day later. Much to our delighted surprise, Da Liu lived just a half block from the Cathedral.

Da Liu, a master with an adventurous and colorful history, became one of my "Rice Paper" teachers (*reference to my first book). He'd begun practicing Tai Chi in 1928 in East-China. Later, during the Japanese occupation, he was forced to leave and emigrated to the Chinese Southeast provinces, where Da Liu studied with many great Taoist, Kung Fu, and Tai Chi masters. Six years after the communist takeover of China, he decided to leave his homeland, this time settling in the U.S., where he became one of only two Tai Chi masters in the country. The other was Chen Man Ching. Both teachers developed what is known as the "short form" of T'ai Chi. Da Liu also taught at the UN's Chinese institute. These two were the first to introduce this subtle Oriental art to the West.

T'ai Chi was the softer form of Kung Fu that had been taught in the Shao Lin temples for a thousand years. Kung Fu itself had evolved from eight trigram boxing–based on principles taught by the Book of Changes, known as the I-Ching.

After Felton Jones and Paul Solomon, Da Liu became my third Rice Paper Teacher.

Wax on / Wax Off

With the Cathedral just a block away, we could take classes twice a week. While Andrew and I made just enough money to pay the rent and buy basic bargain food, we never had $60 a week for our four Tai Chi classes

But Da Liu was agreeable to a work-for-class exchange. I was hired to water his plants and clean his tiny, one-room apartment twice a week. It sounded like a good deal, and it was, but it came with a shock.

I assumed that Da Liu, a Taoist, would have a clean, organized home. I had not yet been to Japan to witness firsthand the cleanliness of Japanese or Chinese Zen Buddhists, roshis, and their Temples, who confirmed the "image" of cleanliness and order associated with Eastern spiritual disciplines.

But no! It was a complete, total mess. This, from a Rice Paper Teacher? The money he had collected from classes was under every book, in the mattress, and scattered everywhere: chaos.

Well, Taoists are not Zen Buddhists. Taoists are Taoists. They study the sayings of Lao Tzu, who wrote about *The Tao Te Ching* ("*The Way*"), devoted to achieving immortality by circulating the Light within us—mysteries further described in the book, *The Secret of the Golden Flower*.

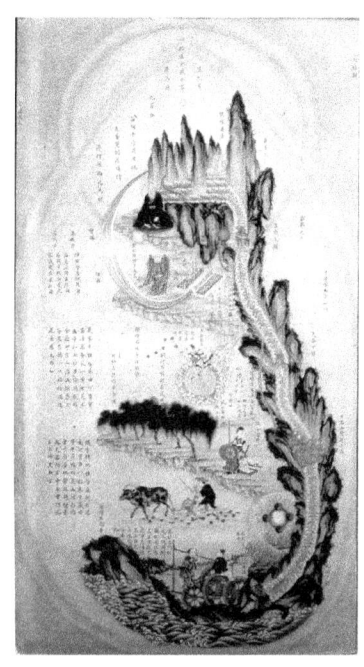

During my studies with him, Da Liu introduced to me **the Neijing tu,** which describes Neidan "Internal Alchemy"— and diagrams internal pathways the Light circulates through the body during the practice of T'ai chi or Taoist meditation.

The original Neijing tu, on the right While the original Neijing tu probably dates from the 19th century (Komjathy 2004:11),all copies derive from an engraved stele dated 1886 in Beijing's White Cloud Temple that records how Liu Chengyin based it on an old silk scroll discovered in a library on Mount Song (in Hunan).

In addition, a Qing Dynasty colored scroll of the Neijing tu was painted at the Ruyi Guan "Palace of Fulfilled Wishes" library in the Forbidden City (Despeux 2008:767).[14]

The origins of Neijing tu are not exact but probably go back to the 13th century A.D. Its depiction of a seated man or fetus in meditation has become popular in Taoist circles. The diagram is a representation of Taoist inner alchemy theory, processes, and techniques. The "map" refers to the practice of the microcosmic orbit (the small Heavenly cycle) of circulating the Light. It clearly shows the process of reversing the flow of the water of life.

---

[14] Wikipedia.

The "chi" or life force is pumped up the spine through three mountain passes to the cranial cavity. The main energy centers, the Tan Tians, otherwise known as the three Elixir fields, are represented in the diagram as the ox, the cowherd, and the old man. Another striking feature is the range of mountain peaks that guide down the universal energy into the center of the brain.

Da Liu never translated the Chinese script on this thousand-year-old painting from the Shao Lin schools. He just pointed to the ancient mapping of the inner course of light when he talked about the *Chi*, our vitality, the light—the power which gives us life. When I pressed him about the meaning of Chinese writing, he didn't respond. I was directed to just practice my Tai Chi "form."

And so I did. I practiced T'ai Chi on the subway platforms waiting for the train to come. I practiced on street corners waiting for the bus. I practiced the T'ai Chi walk, how to open and close doors using T'ai Chi energy, pulling vitality from the ground, through my feet, legs, navel center, and finally pushing on the door with little or no muscular effort.

T'ai Chi was so pervasive; I often dreamed I was doing the "form" and could even do it flying—in my dreams.

I discovered that all I had to do was think "the form," and my hands would get hot from the movement of the Chi.

Da Liu was an industrious writer. Before I arrived, he had already published *The Taoist Health Exercise Book* in 1974. During my apprenticeship with Da Liu in 1980-81, he had asked me if I could help with the English and grammar of his next book project, *T'ai Chi Ch'uan and I Ching: A Choreography of Body and Soul*. He let me correct his English for a few weeks but eventually deemed my writing skills "insufficient" for his taste. Despite my lack of writing skills, he subsequently (1987) published the book and another *T'ai Chi Ch'uan and Meditation* in 1991.

So while my first attempt as a writer and editor fell flat, I still dutifully cleaned his apartment, put his $5, $10, and $20 bills stuffed in books and every nook imaginable in neat piles so that he knew where the money was when he went out to buy his vegetables and his Chinese newspaper every morning. I watered his plants, which had to be watered just right.

He taught balance in all things.

Sometimes we would walk the ten blocks uptown to Columbia University together, where he taught twice a month. During our short trek, he would ask, "Why are we walking this road?" I had no clue. "Because it is shorter and requires less energy to walk," he explained. There was a good Taoist answer to a good Taoist question!

Within just a few months, I was allowed to join the advanced students studying *Push Hands*, a subtle but gentle exercise involving throwing an opponent off balance almost without using any detectable physical energy, and Tai Chi Sword, an exercise using a sword to extend the chi beyond the body.

In eighteen months, I learned what many students took ten years to learn, and Da Liu was quite upset when I suddenly announced that I would be moving back to Hearthfire Lodge. Paul Solomon felt my training under Da Liu was sufficient and that I had reached a level where I could teach T'ai Chi at the school. Billy had moved back to the Lodge a few months before, but it was my decision when I would leave NYC and end my apprenticeship under Da Liu.

It took about a week, but I finally mustered the courage to break the news to Da Liu at his apartment. I had given him no warning about my decision. He was shocked. His eyes flashed a hint of anger, "David, you are leaving just when your form has reached an advanced stage."

I thanked Da Liu for everything he taught me, but they fell like lead paperweights to the floor. I left heartbroken. Da Liu didn't say so, but I felt he'd hoped I'd be his full-time apprentice. But the lessons learned from him were as not forgotten. Enough had soaked in so that I, in turn, in later years, was able to introduce T'ai Chi at Hearthfire to hundreds of Japanese students visiting the Lodge for our 40-day retreat programs.

The teachings of the ancient art of T'ai Chi served to create long life and health for my old friend and master. Da Liu died in 2001, aged 98. It was said that his teacher died at the age of 126. He lived as a Taoist, and he died as a Taoist. Did Da Liu discover the immortal soul he sought to cultivate his entire life?

He was a kind and loving man. I am quite sure he smiled when he walked through the gates of the Jade Mountain.

10

The Faculty

Earth University and the Mystery School

In the 15th century, in a world before telescopes, the Earth was considered motionless, and it was apparent the sun and stars revolved around us. Nicolas Copernicus, the Polish astronomer and priest, had a radical proposal that the Earth was not the center but was just another planet revolving around the Sun. Many took this theory as an affront to Scripture. They were horrified. But one man thought Copernicus didn't go far enough, his name was Giovani Bruno. He was a natural-born rebel. He longed to bust out of this cramped little Universe.

Bruno hungered to know everything about God's creation. He read Copernicus's writings, and that was his undoing. He read Lucretius, the poet and philosopher from the 1st century B.C., who wrote about *the Nature of Things,* whispering to Bruno of a Universe far greater, about a Universe unbounded, about a Universe as limitless, as God. Lucretius asked his readers to stand on the edge of the Universe and shoot an arrow. If it hit a wall, to move to the wall, and shoot another arrow, and so on. If the arrow keeps going, then clearly, that wall must lie beyond what you thought was the edge of the Universe. Then if you stand on that wall and shoot another arrow, and there are only two possible outcomes, one that if it flies forever into outer space or it hits some boundary where you can stand and shoot another one. Either way, the Universe is unbounded.

Bruno realized, at that moment, the Cosmos must be infinite. It made perfect sense, then, that the God he worshipped was infinite. So, he reasoned, how could Creation be anything less?

When he was 30, he had a vision that sealed his fate. He saw a universe as a bowl filled with stars. He experienced a sickening moment of fear as he touched the edge of the bowl to peek underneath. But he summoned up his courage.

"I spread confident wings to space and soared toward the infinite, leaving far behind me what other strained to see from a distance. Here there was no up, no down, no edge, no center. I saw that the Sun was just another Star. And the Stars were other Suns, each escorted by other earths like our own. The revelation of this immensity was like falling in love."[15]

Bruno became an evangelist, teaching *the Gospel of Infinity* through Europe. He thought the other lovers of God would embrace the more comprehensive, glorious view of Creation. He was excommunicated by the Roman Catholic Church in his homeland and by the Lutherans in Germany. He jumped at the chance to lecture at Oxford in England, at last, he thought, an opportunity to share his vision with an audience of his peers. He explained about Copernicus. "They have their own watery Earths, with plants, animals, and man."

The council responded, "Everyone knows there is only one world!"

But Bruno insisted, "Our infinite God has created a boundless Universe *with an endless number of worlds*. Do you not read Aristotle or the Bible? You must reject your limiting beliefs about the Creator. You must *doubt some things to begin anew.*

Your God is too small!

He couldn't keep his vision of an infinite Universe to himself. The penalty in his world was death. Bruno was sentenced to the most vicious form of cruel and unusual punishment and burned at the stake for his views.

---

[15] Giordano Bruno (1548 – February 17, 1600), On the Infinite, the Universe and the Worlds: Five Cosmological Dialogues

There comes a time in our lives that we realize that we are not the center of our universe. With my declining health and early expiration date looming, everything seems centered around my universe, past, present, and future. I want to share some short stories, history, lessons, and aspects of my Earth University and Mystery School experiences. Some are identified by "Wires," which directed and guided the development of my soul.

Carmel-in-the-Valley

Paul Solomon's vision of a Mystery School was not only an ancient Hebrew School, but a blending of Persian, Chinese, Japanese, Hindu, and American Indian Mystery Schools, with great emphasis on Christ. It would include memorization, dream recall, interpretation, and the practice of gardening, bonsai, Tai Chi, and Yoga. All were employed to help a student do what the Apostle Paul admonished all of us to do, renew our mind by donning the Mind of Christ.

In 1977, Paul Solomon and the members of the Fellowship were able to secure a large 1600 acre parcel of land in the Shenandoah Valley and called it Carmel-in-the-Valley. The Master Plan included a carpenter school, a gardening school, a Seminary, a school of music, and a school of healing. It was a massive project. In 1978, Paul Solomon invited Alan Chadwick School of Gardening from Carmel, California. He brought his students and plants and began transforming the property.

Quoted from the Chadwick Legacy Project website, *"Alan arrived with a truckload of plants and greenhouse glass that his dedicated Covelo apprentices had carefully packed for him. The garden quickly took shape under Alan's inspired direction. The transplants thrived.*

In September 1979, when I arrived, I had a chance to hear a few of Alan's lectures at the Carmel property. His Shakespearian background made his lectures dramatic, on the edge of your seat dramas.

Chadwick always taught his students to be stewards of the earth. "We come to the garden unaware of and unmindful of its mysteries, thinking it is just a place where food is produced. In the same way, we think of soil as an inert substance that, thanks to our good fortune, happens to cover enough of the earth's surface to enable us to produce dinner on schedule. We do not perceive the earth as a living thing and that the soil is the skin of the earth." It is a living Being that breathes.

"We have to come back to simplicity, the knowing of the inner senses, all our glands and our nerves, attached to the spinal cord, have a connection to everything that lives in nature; the very wavering of a leaf in the wind, the birth of a seed. It's all a part of us, within us, and in our nerves and glands, like an athlete, the muscles become me effet and extinct. And that is what is happening. We are becoming separated."[16]

Alan's philosophy is that of absolute truth. Absolute simplicity. Absolute purity of heart and intent—especially when approaching the garden. To pirate the land, to put a price on what the earth gives us so freely is to vandalize the land. Neither must we contrive or distort the performance of nature by creating artificiality using hybrid techniques—the word comes from the Greek meaning 'defiance of the will of Heaven.'

---

[16] Quotes from *Reflections of the Inner Light*, March, 1979. pp. 14-15.

Sadly, the continuation of the school collapsed. A large balloon payment was missed, and the Fellowship lost the larger property leaving us with the six-acre lot at Hearthfire Lodge a few miles down the road. Additionally, Alan, at 84, was dying of cancer. The Alan Chadwick School of Gardening returned to the Gulch Zen Center in San Francisco to continue a gardening project. Despite his declining condition, he continued to give lectures until his death in May 1980. [17]." After Carmel, a few of Alan's students remained behind at Hearthfire to teach Alan's world-famous gardening method called *Bio Dynamic, French Intensive gardening.*

Hearthfire Lodge continued to be our little hidden-in-the-woods Mystery School, an Earth University. It was my home. It was my life for 13 years between 1979 and 1992.

Our small parochial school, our little Yeshiva, was just that; a small group of students dedicated a cause. For me, it was always the Spirit of Prophecy that guided the School. I knew we were fast approaching that future time spoken of by Isaiah, by Jesus Christ, and by St. John.. A future described and predicted by all religions, a future that Secular Humanists don't want to talk about, a future that is building around us as we speak, a time spoken of by prophets and the Dead Saints that will occur over the next 20 years.

We were not all ascetics. Some ate fried fish and hamburgers. Many were scholars with their children by their sides, sharing evening meals, cleaning together, and evening study classes. We hosted many well-known world class leaders who flew in from every part of the planet to offer training in their area of expertis. Often Paul Solomon and I would travel to different parts of the world to teach months, which also provided the funds to pay the bills.

---

[17] http://www.talkingchadwick.org/carmel-in-the-valley-new-market-va.html

Paul's international outreach helped create Fellowship Centers in Australia, New Zealand, South Africa, Belgium, Holland, and Japan.

Paul trained ILC (Inner Light Consciousness) teachers to assist him throughout the late 1970s, and 1980's so the burden was not on him alone. During this period, I was his assistant. I shadowed him wherever he went. I watched. I learned. I absorbed. I helped write. I worked with others on our monthly and quarterly Newsletter, laying out by hand-printed script in the days before electronic layout.

In 1979, during my first week's stay at Hearthfire Lodge, Paul Solomon asked me to clean up a nest of spiders on each of the four ceiling corners of the back screened-in porch with a broom. No big deal, but there were hundreds of spider balls nurseries and baby spiders everywhere. I didn't like it one bit. Spiders were crawling all over the place like a house of horrors. It took 30 minutes, but eventually, I swept most of them away. It's something you don't easily forget. I asked myself, why am I doing this, and what is the lesson to be learned?

As I often do now, I check the NDERF.org site to catch up on their weekly NDE updates and found this Dead Saint story from Debbie about loving a spider, I believe, is the crux of our existence. If you can see it, it's one of those training wire lessons that will guide you to a new relationship with love you may never have considered before:

~I had a winter virus with projectile vomiting. Suddenly I could not breathe. I remember thinking, 'Not here, not now.'... When I came out of my body, I was on a bridge. In the distance and over the water was a really beautiful harbor and city infused with a golden light. The feeling of leaning on the side of the bridge, looking at the play of light on the water was an indescribable joy. There were many people milling about the harbor, all who I felt I knew. There were two guides on the bridge with me, which I accepted as normal.

My perspective was strange because I was up in the air, on the bridge, behind myself, and looking at the details of the city and harbor all at the same time.

The guides had two books with them for me to read. The first book was about my life. I could flick through the pages and look at different events, and they helped me judge if they were good or bad. Good decisions were celebrated by the people on the other side of the bridge. The pages were more like films, and I could see how my choices affected everyone around me. I was shocked to find out that a day I had worked hard at the hospice and done my best to help everyone, yet this was celebrated the least by my guides.

The day I helped a spider out of the door was celebrated because I had done it with a feeling of real empathy for the spider despite being afraid of spiders. There was no reward from people knowing what I had done. The message was to do everything with love, which is much tougher than I thought. I became aware that the light around me was conscious and made of pure love. We all belong to this light, and the light is inside us. The guides knew I was curious and let me read the second book. They told me that I would not remember it, and if I tried to, I would possibly misinterpret it. But the book made perfect sense when I was there. The book appeared more like a sphere which represented the cosmos on many different layers and with the loving consciousness permeating endless dimensions and worlds. I remembered everything, but have promised to forget for now...

The experience was profound, and I am still processing it. I do not want to talk to anyone about something as silly as nearly choking to death on my own vomit, so when I have tried to describe the experience, I say it was a dream, and I have not talked to anybody about the two books I saw.[18]

---

[18] *Debbie NDE*, #4097, 03.03.16, NDERF.org

It is not about saving the spider but about making a conscious effort of giving love and expecting nothing in return.

Jesus Christ taught that whoever would be great must become the servant of all. We must learn to become aware of others' needs, to observe their needs, and respond to them. These lessons can only be understood in this Earth University, day to day, experience. It can be accelerated under a teacher's guidance, just as Christ taught his twelve apostles. These lessons include learning or overcoming:

- Letting go of self by thinking of others
- Becoming conscious and mindful of surroundings
- Loving unconditionally
- Learning to follow and obey the "still small voice."
- Learning to receive answers from God.
- Learning to *walk with God*.
  - Telepathic rapport: Learning Line upon Line, Precept upon Precept.

If God were to give a student gifts of the spirit, would the student use them to glorify himself or glorify God? To ensure the latter, teachers emphasized the building of character; your word is your bond in all things. Don't promise what you cannot do. Be accountable for your actions. Most of all, do everything with love. Serve one another.

The Apostle Paul wrote: ~Now if anyone builds on this foundation with gold, silver, precious stones, wood, hay, straw, each one's work will become evident; for the Day will declare it, because it will be revealed by fire; and the fire will test each one's work, of what sort it is. If anyone's work which he has built on it endures, he will receive a reward. 1 Corinthians 3:12- (NKJV)

When we look at the Apostle Paul's statement about the "Day" of Judgment, the day of your life review, it makes sense that the judicial council, You, God, and Jesus, will evaluate your "work." The "fire will burn away" that which is unreal, to reveal that which is real, authentic, and eternal? ~**Chronicle 368**

One lesson I cannot forget; overcoming the fear of fire. In 1982, our little group of students drove to the outskirts of Washington D.C. to take a firewalking workshop hosted by fire walking founder Tolly Burkan.[19] He proposes that firewalking is not a paranormal event but an experience of overcoming fear and encouraging empowerment and healing. Walking over a bed of hot coals has been practiced for over 4000 years globally in many cultures and religions. During the last 40 years, over 3 million Westerners have experienced firewalking. It is often used as a rite of passage to test an individual's strength and courage, or in religion as a test of one's faith. Burkan says,

"Knowing the secret behind firewalking can improve your life. Firewalking demonstrates how your thoughts impact everything else in your life. Thoughts change brain chemistry, and that results in an alteration of body chemistry as well. Firewalkers are instructed to pay close attention to their thoughts since those very thoughts are how we create our realities. Positive thinkers live in a different chemical environment than negative thinkers."

---

[19] Tally Burman is the founder of the international firewalling movement. Tally's approach to firewalling resulted in a global phenomenon of over four million people attending firewalling classes.

In total, about one hundred attended the workshop, seven of us from Hearthfire Lodge. After four hours of team building and creating an atmosphere of "anticipation" (as I remember, trepidation), we all walked outside and gathered in a big circle to watch the big bonfire burn down to coal s, which takes a few hours before it is safe to walk on. As I remember, the firewalk seemed to be nearly twenty-five feet long.

No one was forced to walk the fire plank like a pirate. At the site, I was overwhelmed by the heat from the burning coals to the point that I could tolerate only a fleeting moment within ten feet of the fire pit. And strangely out of the one hundred people—as fate would have it, they raked out a path of coals—directly in front of me.

You walk the coals when you are ready, but it seemed the baton was in my hand to run with. I am unable to explain why I was unafraid. I looked at a spot on the other side of the coals, imagined my Jesus standing there waiting for me.

"I'm in your hands, Lord."

I didn't hesitate. Fate put me in front of the fire to walk first. Before I knew it, I had walked across the burning coal fires to the other side. I felt no great heat or pain. It felt like I was walking on warm cornflakes. As a safety measure, a workshop assistant hosed my feet with cold water if any hot embers might have stuck between my toes. It was over in seconds. No blisters. No tricks. No fear.

After I walked across the hot coals, it triggered the rest of the group to begin walking. All of my classmates made it across. Heck, there were a few twelve-year-olds who walked the fire several times. Once was enough for me! What did I learn?

To have faith and to not be afraid. I didn't see it as a "group building experience" as much as an inner battle to "believe" in a higher power that I would not be harmed.

In early 1982, when Paul Solomon met Chris Van Cleave, who had just completed his second tour of Jesus Christ Superstar. Paul worked on a Rock/Gospel musical for a new Broadway musical called "The Davidson Affair," a story about the return of Jesus Christ to a modern NYC, the gathering of his disciples, and how the world will see Him. The cliff note version of the musical went something like this:

The new administration in Washington has declared that all young men must return to the city of their birth to be registered for the military draft. Due to the economic recession, Josh Davidson and his expectant wife, Maria, have hitch-hiked to New York City so that Josh may register. All New York hotels are over-booked with the influx of registrants and, unable to find a place to stay, Maria goes into labor on a Manhattan sidewalk. A doorman at the Waldorf-Astoria springs into action, taking Maria into the hotel's basement boiler room where Joe Davidson is born. The birth is attended by a taxi-driver (one of the "shepherds" of New York City) and three other "guided" visitors. If the story begins to sound familiar, it should.

It is a potent new telling of the "greatest love story" ever told. It is all too easy to dismiss the relevance of a story that took place 2000 years ago in a very different culture. With the current turmoil in the world and the challenges of our everyday lives, what if a man such as Jesus Christ lived today?

What if he were in your city, sharing his teachings, giving practical advice on how to navigate successfully through these current times? If he taught and demonstrated miraculous healings, showing us we could do all these things and more, would he be condemned and accused of fraud? How would our church and religious leaders respond? Would history repeat itself?

When Paul introduced a new Musical to Chris Van Cleave, Chris dropped what he was doing and began writing music. Within a few days, he wrote the song "Emmanuel," which led to an eighteen-month collaboration between them to create a staged musical *The Davidson Affair*. It was first produced in 1982 for a showcase run of five sold-out performances at the Wells Theater in Norfolk, VA.

During my teenage years, I loved to watch *Jesus Christ Superstar* and *Godspell*. When Paul asked if I wanted to be a part of the Davidson Affair, I jumped at the opportunity. I ended up playing one of the lead roles as the apostle Nathaniel.

I remember one vivid moment during the Musical was the moment of surprise before the packed theater when I realized Joe Davidson 'knew' what I had been doing before we had ever met. Jesus saw Nathanael coming to Him and said of him, "Behold, an Israelite indeed, in whom there is no deceit!"

Nathanael said to Him, "How do you know me?"

Jesus answered and said to him, "Before Philip called you when you were under the fig tree, I saw you."

Nathanael answered Him, "Rabbi, You are the Son of God; You are the King of Israel" Jesus answered and said to him, "Because I said to you that I saw you under the fig tree, do you believe? You will see greater things than these." The audience cracked up at my look of total surprise.

It was a magical moment, indeed. I am such a serious personality that to have a thousand people laugh at me was unforgettable.

After one evening performance, Paul and I were about to leave when a group of Down syndrome teenagers ran up to us in tears to hug us. We spent a few minutes crying and hugging each other. I think that moment of love stands out among one of the most precious I ever experienced.

I was responsible for recording Paul's lectures on reel to reel tape. In late 1981, my Mom, Dad, and sisters followed me up to the Shenandoah Valley to be a part of the School. They lived a few miles down the road in the "Gift Shop," a sound studio called Carmel Voice & Vision, a department Mom initially took over, developing tape catalogs that were advertised in the Supportive Lifestyles Newsmagazine.

My family was only there a year before they moved back to Virginia Beach, at which time, the responsibility was handed over to me. I became the sound engineer and eventually responsible for editing and assembling most of the tape titles and CD sets available today on www.paulsolomon.com.

On October 18, 1983, I was ordained as a minister. Part of my ordination requirements was to complete, along with the assistance of Jennifer S., the Manual for Ordination, a seven-volume Seminary Program guide for all future Fellowship of the Inner Light Ministers.

1984 was a fateful year. Upon our return from Isreal and Greece, Paul felt increasingly ill. Paul had planned to go to Australia to teach a month-long program when he became so sick, sick enough to get some blood work and tests done. When the doctors saw the results, they told him that he wouldn't be returning if he went on a trip like that.

Three days later, after eating a bowl of chili, he woke up in the middle of the night in a lot of pain. Paul was rushed to the hospital and discovered he was critically ill with pancreatitis. We were told he would require emergency exploratory surgery on March 4, 1984; in severe pain, he was rushed to Rockingham Hospital for Emergency surgery. Paul died three times on the operation table. As Paul recounts, the next thing he could remember was that he was dead.

Three times during the surgery, he suffered from cardiac arrest. During each of these episodes, he remembers the same sequence of events. He would leave his body and watch dispassionately as the machine displaying his heart rate flat-lined. As the doctors and nurses frantically worked to defibrillate his heart and get it beating again, he saw around him "angels in shining, resplendent robes with great white wings." He would then find himself walking on a shining path through a tunnel toward a shining city:

Paul Solomon's March 4, 1984 NDE:

I woke up with lights in my face and forms leaning over me. The forms appeared at first to be the faces of beautiful women, but they were transparent. I could see through them, and I knew they were angels.

I reached up to them, threw my arms around them. I hugged them and they hugged me back. Everyone was transparent. They were light beings, and I saw only light, no flesh, and they all let me hug them.

As I began to become more conscious, if that is the word, they became more solid and it seemed sad. As I became more deeply ingrained in the flesh, I saw flesh. I realized that they were doctors and nurses, and as I began to see flesh, I began to feel pain.

When I was in spirit, in light, and little aware of the flesh, I saw light. I knew the light was still there when I could no longer see it, and it helped to remember that as the nurses would cane and go. Each time I would see their faces, I would remember that night and the light that I saw in them, and I would try to see it again and remember it whether I could see it or not.

I began to remember what had happened and what I was doing there laying in that hospital bed with tubes in every opening in my body, and same in newly cut openings.

I had planned to go to Australia to teach a month long program, when I started to feel sick, sick enough to tests. When the doctors saw the results, they told me that if I went on a trip like that I wouldn't be caning back. I asked the Source of my guidance what to do, and the response was that it was no more dangerous to go to Australia than to stay at home, so I had decided to go, but I never went.

It was three days later that I woke up in the middle of the night with a lot of pain. I knew I'd better go to the hospital. I remember them telling me they were going to do exploratory surgery, and I was too sick to do anything but agree.

The next thing I remember, I was dead. God was saying to me with a rather familiar voice, "You can make a decision. You can go on now or you can stay, but if you stay, you have to take a whole new step in this work."

"God, I can't make the decision. I just don't want to deal with that decision," I said.

And so God said, "We'll put you on hold."

When I woke up from the experience with doctors and nurses and around me, they told me that I had died twice that night. I had been pronounced clinically dead.

After Paul recovered from his NDE at Rockingham Hospital in Harrisonburg, Virginia, he was transferred to the University of Virginia hospital. I packed my bags, drove behind the ambulance, and walked him through admissions until he was assigned a room.

This began my "Nursing Wires."

I spent the next three months with him in the hospital from 8:00 a.m. to 10 p.m. Exploratory surgery at Rockingham revealed acute pancreatitis, one of the most painful diseases known. The golden treatment for acute pancreatitis was to pump his stomach every day, so stomach fluids did not excite the pancreas.

Paul was essentially forced into a 40 day fast by the minute by minute removal of these stomach fluids. To start the process, the nurse threads a plastic tube through the nose, down to the stomach, to begin the stomach pumping process emptied into a clear plastic container.

The next step was to thread another plastic tube directly into Paul's heart. This tube was to feed liquefied vitamins and nutrition directly into the heart, the only artery large enough to handle infusion acidity. The reality of inserting the tube was one of the most painful procedure you can imagine. As the doctor began threading the tube, Paul writhing in pain, a passing nurse looked in, saw his agony, rushed into his room, ran over to him, and held his hand.

She stared directly at the ceiling in passionate prayer, and her face was shown as an angel. Tears running down his face, Paul turned to her and smiled, "The pain is gone." "God bless you. God bless you," he said over and over again.

Days were not without humor. One afternoon he fell asleep and began eating an imaginary cheeseburger in slow motion. It was hilarious. He said Gandhi in a dream visited him, and they had a great conversation about fasting. Of course, I never heard either side, but I can only imagine they had a good chat.

During the three months at the hospital, I still brought Paul the Washington Post religiously every morning, and toward the end, the Folgers instant coffee. The life of a student never ends.

I drove Paul back to Hearthfire Lodge in June 1984. Paul never was the same after that. His Dead Saint description of God putting him on "hold" appeared precisely that. On-Hold. For three years. I was his nurse-aide, managing all medicines and insulin for Type II diabetes. I gave him insulin twice a day. I cooked his meals. He booked a few lectures here and there. But it was not the same.

That changed in 1987. Paul was contacted by Makoto A., a small spiritual study group based in Hitachi-Shi, two hours north of Tokyo. They had 15 Japanese students interested in taking our 40-day Mystery School Synthesis Program during the spring of 1987. It sparked new life in Paul. Not only a new life, he decided to marry Sharon, a long time committed student and close friend of Paul. They tied the knot in the summer of 1987. It was a grand, black top hat wedding.

It poured all day! I mean cats and dogs.

I remember wondering, "Paul, why marry now?" "Did God take you off hold?" I sat back and watched, curious about how his life would play out from here. He was choosing to move along a different path. It changed everything for me.

Now that Paul married Sharon, a new path lay before me. It was time to begin removing some of my soul's training wires to unveil a maturing Bonsai.

The Fold

Temple Wires: Priests, Bonsai and Temple Teachers

~When I lived in Japan, I once met a Buddhist priest who so loved King David that when he was a teenager, he bought a clay bust of the King, smashed it up, and ate it so the spirit of David would live inside him. His name is Sugasawa san. ~Chronicle 388

TAMO-SAN

The Japanese "contingent," as I called them (see photograph), led to our first visit to Japan in early February 1987. Emiko arranged for Paul Solomon and me to travel to Japan, where we were met with a whirlwind of television, public lectures, and an introduction to Tamo-san, Emiko's Teacher, the first recognized enlightened Buddhist priestess in 500 years.

I traveled with Paul Solomon throughout Japan, and Emiko was our translator and interpreter. We were hosted on many major Japanese television shows. We became popular. We couldn't travel by subway without someone pointing at us, recognizing us from the TV, it was quite strange. The Japanese people love everything related to psychics. With Paul Solomon being known as the second Edgar Casey, they were quite excited. I ended up conducting offer 300 Paul Solomon source readings in Japan, mostly done at the home of Makoto Asano, but Readings were done at Tamo san's Temple in Kamakura, Japan.

By the way, the traditional picture of the Japanese boarding a bullet train for a 2-hour ride is real. When the doors open, like the old school days of grabbing a seat on the school bus before there are none left. People shoving to get a seat is real. You had to move fast to get a seat, of course, in deference to the elderly.

You wanted a seat, so you would not have to stand for the two hour trip to Kamakura, Tamo san's Temple.

After Paul's marriage to Sharon at Hearth Fire Lodge, Paul and I discussed my marital options. We discussed who might be the ideal "wife" for me, an arranged marriage, like in the old days. Emiko and I had gotten close during her stay at Hearthfire Lodge in 1987 when she was a translator for the Japanese group who travel from Japan to spend 40 days in retreat. Paul and I believed that a spiritual marriage between Emiko, Tamo san's student, and me, Paul's apprentice, was perfect. So the wedding was set.

This same year I moved to Japan with Emi. I traveled with her at all times, not only because she was a professional interpreter and translator and in charge of everything Japanese, but we were engaged to be married in April the following year.

Returning to Tamo san's temple, it was a chilly, sunny afternoon. The ides of October brought out the intense orange, yellow, and reds of the Japanese maples in the city by the sea. Reaching the Shinto temple entrance, we walked under the traditional clay-roof entrance into a Heavenly garden filled with Japanese maples, bamboo, and azaleas dotted throughout the courtyard. Completely enclosed by six-foot-high walls, the temple grounds were pathed throughout by specially selected granite stones spaced in-between with moss, laid out carefully among the trees, bushes, and plants—all creating mystical tranquility you felt in your soul.

There in the garden, we found the slender priestess in rose-colored kimono robes weeding her garden. At 80-years-old, Tamo san stood a young 5'1" tall for a Japanese Buddhist priestess in the land of the Rising Sun.

Tamo san walked up and gave a strong bear hug, lifting me off the ground upon seeing us. Can you imagine? I was only 170 pounds at the time, but her strength was amazing for her slight frame and age. She told me people with few problems are easy to lift, and thank God I was easy!

Tamo san led us to the temple entrance, rolled open the white shoji screen doors to the temple interior, revealing a large open space and a breathtaking view of the main sanctuary and altar. We walked together through the opening, slipped off our shoes, and walked onto the soft bamboo tatami mats covering the floor.

The sanctuary was similar to most Christian monasteries, with an altar on one end. Instead of wooden benches for worshippers, the wall to wall tatami mat bamboo floor was Zen simple – no cushions or chairs. Three steps to a raised platform led to a beautifully ordered altar, one simple candle, and fruit baskets to receive donations from visitors to the temple. Adorned on either side of the altar wall were two six-foot scrolls artfully painted in black Japanese Kanji, translated they read, "The Wisdom of Inner Light." Tamo san says the "light of wisdom" is everywhere, in every place, without limits.

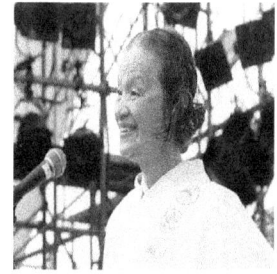

Born Ryoju Kikuchi in 1908, Tamo san was the third child of a Buddhist priest. When she reached the age of twenty-two, she prepared for ordination in the Nishi Hongangii Temple of the Jodo-Shinshu Buddhist sect.

While waiting in the room before the ceremony, she gazed at a rice paper scroll on the wall that read, *Seeing the Truth.*

Then something miraculous occurred. As Tamo san stared at the kanji calligraphy, the scroll broke into millions of golden white particles and streamed into her body. During her mystical-death experience, she saw the universe's birth and how the universe is made of light. She realized the cosmos, nature, and humans appear separate from one another; they are inseparable.

In Buddhism, she touched the periphery of what Buddhists call "Buddha Nature." Buddhists define this illuminated state, "The core, the seed, the trunk, the foundation, and the root of all that exists."

It is familiar because we could apply the same definition of "Buddha nature" to Christian descriptions of the Light described by St. John: 1-5: *"In the beginning was the Word, and the Word was with God, and the Word was God. The same was in the beginning with God. All things were made by him; and with him was not anything made that was made. In him was life; and life was the light of men. And the light shineth in darkness; and the darkness comprehended not."*

Within a year, Tamo san left the Hongangii Temple and traveled for ten years all over Japan and other countries to preach and write. She published her notable work, *Moor the Boat*, an admonishment to humankind that we begin caring for our Mother Earth, lest human disasters destroy the planet. Her love for nature eventually led her followers to call her Tamo san, which means *first mother*.

I wrote some of my first impressions of Tamo san November 21st, 1987 to Paul Solomon:

"She has no fear and sees only the light in others. Her eyes are as clear as glass. She walks with the eagerness of a young child. Her body is hot, even though the air is cold. I could never have imagined a woman of 80 years could be as strong as she or as preserved, if I may use that word, as she. Even though her face is wrinkly, her body is like a young baby, as smooth as silk.

She sleeps only two to three hours a night. Tamo spends her nights writing and meditating on thoughts, she says, that well-up from inside her. Tamo walks through her temple with a child-like grin on her face all the time. When she saw me she told me many wonderful words of inspiration in Japanese! I couldn't understand a word she was saying. Emi is not always present to interpret, yet Tamo speaks to me anyway. Can you imagine? What do you do? I feel silly standing there so helpless.

It's late November now, and most of the time, the weather stays reasonably warm during the day, but the nights are cold. The temple has no heat, so I am painfully learning how to manage my body temperature in the cold air at night. Even though I wear long underwear and a jacket, I still feel cold! My first night, I slept in all my clothes. Tamo san, of course, wears only a long sleeve thin silk kimono. It's very thin but apparently warm enough! When I am cold, she says, "I am hot!" and takes off her top kimono cover.

Her daughter, Shizuru, spends much of her free time away from work to visit her mother, and make sure she is alright. Kanai sensei cooks the most amazing Japanese meals. Every meal Tamo san sits with us to eat. Lunch and dinner consist of vegetables and white rice. Sometimes fried tofu and miso soup. Tamo picks wild weeds from her garden for our daily salad. The idea, she says, is that weeds will grow in the garden which our bodies need to stay healthy. Some weeds will appear when our bodies get sick, so it's important to notice when they appear in the garden, so we can pick them for our salad. Tamo says if we eat the mixture of 15 wild weeds, our bodies will become like new in seven to nine years.

Tamo san has attempted to make her body, life and home a perfect example of nature itself. It is as if she were the incarnation of the Spirit of Nature.

'She was pure, wise, and bright. She calls the Light in Nature, kami (God). I see no difference between God's Light in Tamo san, and the Light of Jesus Christ. She has a quality to her presence similar to the presence I experienced in 1981, when I met Christ in guise of a bag lady on 92nd and Broadway, in New York City.'

The quiet of the temple weighs gently on my mind. I didn't realize this until I left the temple grounds for a few days to apply for a job teaching English in Tokyo. I felt such a peace and calm. My body felt softer. My mind felt, what can I say, gentle? At night my dreams are becoming alive, unbelievably vivid."

Tamo san's teachings were very simple. Be happy, there is no reason not to be. Eat naturally and drink pure water. She said, "You are surrounded by beauty. Everything glows with brilliant light and we are all part of the same Being called Nature. All we need to do is to see things with the eyes of God, a gift we all possess."

All we need to do is to see things with different eyes, which all of us possess. Thus, Butsugen (the eye of God) is what we need to open up within ourselves. After that happens, everything will return to its natural order and until then, suffering will continue to exist.

She says, "The mistake of mankind began when he believed the sun was his only source of light. There is a pure light of wisdom that shines, that casts no shadow."

Message from *Moor the Boat* [20]

Dear friends, you are worried about the threats of war or concerned over the use of nuclear energy, both these problems are certainly very serious. You should, however, be aware that mankind is faced with far graver problems.

---

[20] http://moortheboat.wholelifewholeworld.com/about-Tamo san/through-the-eyes-of-the-enlightened/

If you should come to realize those graver problems, you would be surprised to discover that the good old days have long since passed, the good old days when mankind could afford to worry about the threats of war.

Unless mankind can see the extreme seriousness of the true problem, humanity cannot make any steps towards any brighter destiny, even if the war threats could be rooted out and the problems of nuclear energy be solved. The problems of war threats and nuclear energy concern merely the internal affairs of the group of any kind, or, so to say the driftwood, but have nothing to do with the crucial plight of the driftwood that is carrying the entire ant kind, which keeps on running headlong towards the waterfall, regardless of war or peace aboard it.

If though, least probable, the war threats should be eliminated once and for all, mankind as a whole would still be heading every day to their doom. Some believe that the recent progress in medical science has made the man's life longer, but the individual human longevity is one things and the longevity of mankind itself is another. The doomed fate of mankind would not slow down its pace, whatever agreement may be reached among the people of the world, should we fail to do something about mankind's march towards the waterfall. [21]

According to Tamo san, the first thing we must do is to moor the drifting boat of mankind to the river bank and thus to insulate it from the dangerous cataract:

Tamo san continues:

One may imagine a sight of billions of ants on board a piece of driftwood, floating on a fast-running stream. The ants are apparently, unaware that their driftwood is nearing a cataract. They seem to be even ignorant of the fact that they are on the driftwood.

---

[21] Tamo San (Ryoju Kikuchi) 1981. *Moor the Boat*. Chapter 1.

If they were aware, how could they afford to hate one another, scheme against one another, or be occupied with greed and hostility? The moment when their driftwood falls down the cataract, what would anything mean to one or another ant, friend or foe? This pathetic sight is nothing but an epitome of today's mankind.

She says, 'There is only one choice left in order that mankind should escape this plight. That is, the whole mankind must come reunited into one whole being-unity and cope with the task for readiness. This task is far beyond the capacity of any one nation, any one organization, any one ideology or any one religion.'[22]

We need to begin living on 1/3 less than our current income, because the future economic crash will require we live with less money, food, and heat. We cannot love someone we really hate. We must develop a compassion and understanding for other people that comes from deep inside." It is strange we have laws forbidding killing when we allow killing in war. War makes killing lawful and it violates natural law.

Unfortunately, people see the ideal to be clear, but how to reach the ideal is another matter. Tamo san told me, that it will take time for all of mankind to be awakened, but when it happens, it happens to all of us simultaneously. The darkest time of the day is right before dawn. Now is the dark time, so the dawn is near.

Tamo san was fifty years ahead of her time. She saw an ecological disaster coming, a 6th Extinction coming.[23]

An immediate response is needed to solve world economic, political, and environmental problems. We don't have time to wait for another generation of children to solve our problems. If we don't stop burning fossil fuels, the polar ice caps will melt.

---

[22] Ibid. chapter 1.
[23] The Sixth Extinction

She says the Greenhouse Effect resulting from additional carbon dioxide gases will happen very, very fast. Mankind, she says, is like a pest that eats all the leaves of a tree, and at last, when too many leaves are destroyed, the tree dies. Earth is a tree, and it will not be long before her leaves are gone, causing the earth to die.[24]

Regarding religion, Tamo says, "To make another religion or organization wrong is a hell that binds us to a belief created by human minds, and thus the earth is filled with hell and the prisons of hell. She further asks, "Why is it that humanity has been unable to establish the criterion of telling the good from the evil, or the right from the wrong, after thousands of years of endless arguments to label good and bad. How can we now approach this mystery of standards that all are judged by?"[25]

Tamo continued, "The universe itself is a living existence. Every part is like a cell in one body. Kill one cell, and the whole body knows it. All living and non-living beings, animals, plants, rocks are equally precious. Along with mankind, they have a right to be here. We believe we are separate beings, but we are one being. If we know we are one; we will not want to fight. Why would we fight ourselves?"

This "one cell" connectedness is universal to the NDE and not restricted to religious belief. Mohammad, a Muslim, was 26 when he had a head-collision while driving on a rough road 300 miles south of Tehran in 1977. He was brought to a hospital in unbearable pain where the doctors and nurses started working on him right away. Suddenly, "everything shifted," and he felt a deep calm and peace engulf him:

"When I was a ten, I had bullied and mercilessly beaten another boy who was also around my age. He felt tortured and deeply hurt. In my life review, I saw that scene again.

---

[24] Ibid. chapter 1.
[25] Tamo San (Ryoju Kikuchi) 1981. Moor the Boat. Chapter 3.

The boy was crying in physical and deep emotional pain. As he was walking in the street crying and going back home, he radiated negative energy which affected everything around him and on the path. People and even birds, trees, and flies received this negative energy from him, which kept propagating throughout the Universe. Even rocks on the side of the street were affected by his pain. I saw that everything is alive and our way of grouping things in categories of 'alive' and 'not alive' is only from our limited physical point of view.

In reality everything is alive. I felt all of the pain and hurt that I had inflicted upon him inside of myself. When this boy went home to his parents, I saw the impact that seeing him in that state had on his parents. I felt the feeling and pain it created in them and how it affected their behavior from that point forward. I saw that as a result of this action, his parents would be always more worried when their son was out of home or if he was a few minutes late.

I saw that whenever I had done something good to anyone or anything, that I had done it to myself. And whenever I had hurt someone, I had done it to myself while actually doing that person a favor because they would receive some form of compensation or help from the Universe as a result. This universal gift would be bigger than the damage I had caused to them."[26]

Tamo-san led a simple life, spending her days weeding her garden and nights writing on rice paper, sleeping only two or three hours at night. We had many stays at the Temple between 1987 and 1991, and while my Japanese never really grew beyond five-hundred words, I learned from her an essence of tranquility and love.

---

[26] Mohammad Z NDE, 3991, .08.14.15, NDERF.org

One profound experience with Tamo san happened during my second tour of Japan after I married Emiko. We walked into the kitchen area and sat down to eat slices of sweet persimmon she had prepared for us. My visit to the garden Temple was one of many, but today was different. Paul Solomon had asked me to deliver a special gift to Tamo san, a 24" heavy, brass Crucifix to adorn her Inter-faith altar. When I pulled the Crucifix from the bag and placed it on the kitchen table, Tamo san's eyes opened wide, not out of gratefulness, but out of horror. She screamed and ran out of the kitchen!

Shocked, we didn't know what to do. Of course, only knowing a few words of Japanese, I felt helpless. Emi waited about thirty minutes before pursuing her. Tamo san returned as tears rolled down her face as she spoke to Emi in Japanese while I listened. Translating, Emi turned to me and asked if we could take Jesus off the Cross. Screws held our Lord to the Crucifix, so it was easy to remove them in short order. Tamo san held out her hands to gently receive the brass effigy and caressed Him like a child for what seemed an hour. Every time I relive this moment, I break down and cry. The love she exhibited for the brass image of Christ just blew me away. The moment was so precious. She appeared to be in some internal dialogue with the universe I could not see, hear, or understand.

Eventually, she stood up, holding the brass Jesus in her hands as if He were a baby child. She motioned to me to bring the Cross and follow her to the altar in the main sanctuary. Emi and I walked across the tatami mats to the beautiful central altar area, where Tamo san pointed to an empty spot next to a two-foot brass Buddha, where she ceremoniously placed the Cross. Still holding Jesus, Tamo san lovingly and carefully laid Him at the base of the Cross. She told Emi to stand Jesus upright to indicate *He was a Living Christ, not a Crucified Jesus.*

Every time I read this, it brings me to tears. It was an unforgettable experience I will cherish all my life. The upright Jesus at the foot of the brass cross remained next to Buddha in Tamo san's temple.

Tamo san encouraged Emi and me to experience waterfall purification. She must have known I had a fear of cold and ice. At first, I didn't want to go. Ice cold water scared me to death, so the thought of sitting in my underwear— pitch black darkness— for five to ten minutes under a 37-degree waterfall, seemed a bit extreme to me.

I sighed and agreed to make the trip to the nearby mountains where there was a Japanese hot spring retreat, complete with lodging and good Japanese food. We all walked in heavy white robes about a half-mile to the falls. I could hear their roar before I saw them. One by one, we lined up, peeled off our warm robes, and stepped barefooted into the ice-cold water, and waded over and carefully seated ourselves on a rock under the waterfall. When it came to my turn, I don't remember much—except for the moment when I sat on the rock, slammed my hands together in prayer, and let the heavy force of the snow water pelt over my head and shoulders. It felt like snow slush. I think the shock of the cold water numbed my skin to the point that I began to feel warm. I prayed and prayed and prayed. I think I prayed harder for the water torture to end. It was strangely timeless. I think the whole point of the waterfall purification experience is to focus on God while risking your life.

I don't know how long I was under the waterfall, but at some point, I peeled myself away and stumbled to shore for the warmth of my robe. When everyone finished, we began the half-mile march back to the hot spring Lodge. Before we left, I slipped on an icy rock and stepped back into the freezing water, soaking my tennis shoes.

I never imagined how much pain ice water-soaked tennis shoes could cause during the half-mile walk back to the lodge. I distinctly remember saying to myself, "This is not spiritual"—complaining all the way back, where thank God, I got relief from my agonizing feet in a hot sauna bath.

Emiko asked me if I wanted to go early the next morning. I told her, "maybe." I wrestled with appearances. I didn't want to be the American who was "afraid." Later that night, I dreamed about bees stinging and chasing me. Suffice to say, when she woke me to go through another round of waterfall training, I declined to go.

Ice cold water and bees. At least I gave the waterfall experience a go. The bee test would come years later when yellow jackets attacked me at Akio, my garden home in Washington.

Tamo san passed away on November 21, 2001, at 94. As Emiko recalls, "There were ten of us seeing her off that morning. When she passed, the room filled with a golden light consisting of golden particles, which most of us saw.

Bonsai study with Takanohashi Sensei

It was an hour's ride by train ride to Tokyo to Takanohashi sensei home.

You could not tell from looking outside his home that he had terraced landscaping Japanese kingdom behind he had many granite stones filled with ferns and moss, in a pathway that led to the back of his home. Opening the old cedar gate, I walked into a kingdom of several hundred bonsai masterpieces. Takanohashi sensei loved all different types of azaleas.

Before entering the garden, we would greet his wife. Walking through the back door, we had to remove our shoes. Most traditional Japanese homes have bamboo tatami mat floors. Ms. Takanohashi met Emiko and me at the door, bowed in old Japanese style from her waist to her head to the floor, and deference to her husband and guests. This ancient tradition is not practiced as often by the younger, new generation of Japanese. She served hot green tea and red bean sweets and rice crackers, which by now you can tell, is a staple snack offering for all visitors.

Today, Takanohashi displayed a 700-year-old YEW; he inherited from his Bonsai teacher decades before, about 2.5 feet high by 3.5 feet wide. This particular tree this particular Bonsai tree and one many awards for its beauty and perfection. I wish I had a picture to show you, but back in 1988, we didn't take a lot of photographs.

Bonsai training sessions would start after tea and snacks, but then the training began in his Bonsai Gardens, which were terraced on three levels. The teacher did not speak any English at all. Emiko would help translate, but often it was showing tell, and they would say "ko, ko, ko," which means do it this way, do it this way, do it this way.

My training started with a young specimen, a Japanese white pine. We began with coiling copper wire, not aluminum, around the branches, starting at the bottom and working upwards to the tree's apex. Every branch had to be wired. At the very least, it was an eight-hour wiring process; my fingers would become very sore. It was a tedious job.

Different gauges of wire were used depending on the thickness of the branch. The main branches were first. I had to be aware of the direction the wire would be wound because if wound the wrong way when bending a branch and loosened; it meant I had to rewire the branch in the opposite direction—quite a pain.

It was the mastery of not wiring too tightly or too loosely, or in the wrong direction.

Over 18 months, I learned soil mixtures, style, planting, and transplanting trees and trim the spring growth candles (rabbits and turtles). There are many pieces to bonsai training, including soil mixture's planting styles, lilting techniques to create Nebari, ROOTS, which show the character of a Bonsai Tree. And to know the showman, the Front of a Bonsai Tree. There are air layering techniques, so if a Bonsai Tree has poor Nebari, I could "air layer" the trunk by tightening the wire around its trunk, cover it with wet Sphagnum moss, which forced the Bonsai tree to grow new roots. It was frankly quite impressive.

Takanohashi sensei practiced many different bonsai styles from literati style to cascade style o forest style, formal uprights, semi cascades, and cascades. Sometimes he brought in trees from the wild and explained that it might take many years of cutting one root at a time before he could remove the entire tree from its mountainside sett. Patience. Patience. Patience.

Sensei would have never become a bonsai master if he had not got up at 4:30 every morning to water, fertilize, train, prune, and wire his trees. He had a job; he left at 6:30 for the company job, which paid for his living. I noticed about the Japanese people that if you wanted to be and do something more significant than the average person, you had to get up two hours early to do it because everybody worked.

At one point, he became confident enough about my Bonsai skills that he took me with him to a local college where I demonstrated to the students there how to wrap wire and to create a style from a young bonsai Yew. In the end, he grunted in approval like a proud Mr. Miyagi.

He died at age 74, not long after I left. I never knew he was ill. He was a very compassionate man, always smiling. He loved his bonsais' like his children. I don't know what happened to his bonsai after he died, but I can only imagine they were donated to museums and other places of honor that he deserved. It is obvious he was a rice paper teacher, a master of an art craft.

Even though we only spent a year and a half together, we developed a special bond, a bond that never goes away. In many ways, our relationship was like that of the Karate Kid, except he spoke no English, and I spoke no Japanese. And that is why I use the bonsai azalea tree on the front of this book to show my respect and affection. The tree shows the roots, the beautiful Nebari, which he would love most, much like his azalea bonsai.

So it was my teacher, who had passed, came to me in a dream, to help me and let me know he was really alive.

While in Japan, I had also spent two-years teaching girls high school English. They're just like American girls; they often do not do their homework.

I loved everything Japanese. I learned hiragana and the romaji. It was at least enough to read the romanized version of congee, which can be spoken in languages both in Chinese and Japanese. The words I learned, the 500 words, I still remember today. I wish I could've become fluent in Japanese. It's one of those bucket list things that now I've run out of time to do maybe another time.

Because of the language barrier, I often would watch sumo wrestling, eagerly wait for the 6 o'clock NHK news.

Breakfast every morning at Emiko's home with her family, mother, brother, and sister. Her mother always cooked breakfast. Every day we had a thin white fish seared brown, white rice and an over-easy egg, and vinegar grated cabbage. It was the same every morning, and it was lovely. Everybody would start talking in Japanese, and I would always only catch a few words here, but my mind would drift off.

In the dining room, a Shinto and Buddhist altar sits a few feet below the ceiling adorned with a miniature Temple, dedicated to their ancestors, those family members who have died before them. Nearly every Japanese home has one. In many ways, I felt very much like Gandhi and his little interfaith community in India among the Japanese. Buddhists, Shinto priests, or any Japanese person of faith never saw my Christian beliefs as a barrier to discuss God or Jesus Christ. They wanted to integrate Christians' beliefs but were confused when the Christians refused to consider and integrate Buddhist and Shinto beliefs, which they found very strange.

The dining room and kitchen were the only heated rooms in the house, typical for a Japanese home. So if it got down to freezing at night, the rest of the house was freezing. Typically, one sitting at a table that had a heat lamp underneath which would heat the legs and if it was cold above you could see your breath. It was that cold we always had a bowl of fruit and ripe, bright orange persimmons which Emiko would cut up along with red bean sweets and rice crackers. You can't imagine how many types of red beans sweets there are in Japan. Emiko's brother loved to go out and drink at night, and we had Sochi and sake. And again, you can imagine how many types of Sochi and Sake choices you have in Japan, much like we have thousands of red and white wine choices in the US.

There's a wonderful new movie called *The Birth of Sake,* a documentary of an old-style sake brewing company, which specializes in making Sake from scratch in the old ways.

There were many wonderful experiences in Japan, it was not all work. We had a chance to travel over many months to many of the sacred Temples throughout Japan.

Through Makoto Asano, we met Sugasawa san on Mount Kōya, Japan, the birthplace of Kūkai (空海), (also known as Kobo Daishi.).[27] Japan's countryside is spectacular, especially during the fall with the beautiful leaves and the steam baths. It is something like out of the 19 century when you walk down the street in a kimono, going to a restaurant to eat sushi; it is an experience. You have to feel to understand what it is like; you cannot imagine.

An interesting piece of information is that when the United States decided which cities to drop the nuclear bombs during World War II, they wanted to avoid the temples in Osaka and the other cities not to destroy the ancient temples. After the atomic bombs were dropped on Japan, Tamo san went to the emperor and advised him to surrender to the United States forces immediately. Such was the clout Tamo san had with the Emperor.

I hope this paints a picture for you of my time in Japan, what it was like to bend and sometimes remove my soul's training wires. After a few years in Japan, Emiko and I returned in 1992 to the US to live in a small apartment in Virginia Beach. The move to the U.S. brought difficulties in our marriage; my own flawed relationship decisions ended our marriage in 1993.

We remain friends. There are so many experiences that happened in Japan. I could write another book about it. For now, it is enough.

---

[27] Wikipedia: Kaia (空海), also known as Kobo Daishi, Founder of Shingon, Buddhism. Born 774 – died 835. (age 61). Zentsūji, Sanuki Province, Japan.

―― 12 ――

The Firm

Enterprise Wires

An unknown Dead Saint writes: God gave me a message and sent me home. He said, 'You must tell the people. You must tell the people to stop going for the diamond and settle for the brass. Families who go for the diamond are workaholics, parents don't know their children, and children don't know their parents. Families are breaking apart everywhere. You MUST tell them to stop going for the diamond. 28 ~

When Paul Solomon died suddenly in early March 1994, I fell into an emotional tailspin. When I was dating my ex-wife and discovered the same day as his Memorial Service, she was pregnant with our son, Benjamin. We married in late September, bought a condo on October 1, just in time for Benjamin's birth on October 15th. For income, I worked as a car salesman at the local Checkered Flag auto dealership. My dream still was to complete my two-year research for the book tentatively titled, The Final Judgment, a title I later changed to The Armageddon Stones. I hoped to devote myself entirely to the project, but the need to make a living always interfered.

I contacted my now ex-wife and asked for her help to raise funds to complete my "comet book" project. We were still friends, and she always laughed at my "comet epiphany" in her house in Japan. One of our mutual friends, Akito, made a generous donation, and soon I began researching (before Google) for Biblical, geological, and paleontological evidence for comet impacts in recent history.

---

[28] (Unknown NDERF.org quote reference)

I spent the next twelve months traveling to London, Wisconsin, and Washington DC, researching the first draft of my book when I ran out of funds. My son was only a year old, and I had bills to pay. The Fellowship was a small church with no paid pastor positions available. I had no job to fall back on.

I had to do something--I just didn't know what. I still have yet to get them published and hope to get Akito a copy of the book as he desired that it would be done. (2020 – It is still to be published.)

Early that summer, 1995, my wife saw a local commercial about building your own home business and suggested we listen to a lecture at the Cavalier Hotel in Virginia Beach. I told her that all those business opportunities were scams and didn't want to go. She dragged me to the lecture anyway, and wouldn't you know it; I was the first to pay $2000 on a credit card to learn all about selling distressed merchandise, kind of an early version of Overstock.com.

Yep, it was a scam, but I didn't know it yet.

The business opportunity offered group buying power to obtain distress merchandise at wholesale prices and sell it at a profit. We got set up for business; computers, copier, fax/phone, and an inventory of distressed merchandise to sell; cameras, jewelry, and electronic equipment. In 1995, marketing was done mostly by fax, brochures, or call center. The internet, for all practical purposes, was still a few years away.

We got a merchant account set up to accept credit cards like any regular business. In those days, we used software that made your computer into a credit card terminal for authorization and batching out at the end of the day. It was like magic, seeing your money settle into your business checking account in 48 hours.

We sold a few items here and there for a couple of months over the summer, but we quickly discovered our investment far exceeded our profits. We promptly went thousands of dollars into debt, and most of it on credit cards to support the business.

I am not one to give up easily. I paid another $2000 to get "coached" on how-to-do the distressed Fax business even better. I discovered the coach in Salt Lake City personally coached nearly sixty people a week, and altogether twenty other coaches coached over 2000 people a week. And I found they all needed to accept credit cards to sell their distressed stuff.

Then, I had a crazy idea. I contacted a local credit card processor in Virginia Beach. I told him about the business coaches in Salt Lake City who needed to get merchant accounts setup for merchants in the distressed merchandise fax business. He told me he would pay me $50 a referral. I thought, wow. I could make more money getting referrals than selling stuff. I was paid for a few weeks, and then suddenly, the referral money stopped, and calls to find out why went unreturned. Did he go around me and talk directly to the coaches in Salt Lake City?

One night, while soaking in a hot tub, debating what to do about it, I had an epiphany. I thought, "What if I get a job for the company in Salt Lake and have instant access to all the coaches in the building? And at the same time, what if I get trained to learn the credit card business and bring on these merchants myself? I realized there was much more than $50 per merchant to be made.

Move to SLC

I flew to SLC the next week to speak with the company's owners about moving from Virginia Beach to become a coach in their company.

They liked the idea and told me they would hire me when I arrived. They offered to pay me $3000 a month, which was $3000 more than I was making at the time.

So with that verbal nod, we abandoned our newly purchased condo, packed everything we owned in a U-Haul, and moved to Salt Lake City.

When I arrived a few days later (my wife and my baby had flown out ahead of me), I parked the U-Haul truck in the parking lot and marched up to the administration office to announce my arrival. I met the owner who looked at me like, "Who are you?" He didn't even remember talking to me a week before. "We don't have any openings available." Incredulous, I threw the paper pad I was carrying to the floor in front of him and said, "I just moved my family in a U-Haul two-thousand miles on your word I had secured a job here. Not only that, I am the only coach who knows how to sell this stuff. I've done it. You need me." I didn't yell. And I don't remember exactly how I presented myself, but I had a kid and a wife in the car, and I had no way to rent an apartment. If I failed here, I most likely would have to move back to Virginia Beach.

The company boss stared at me for a moment and told me to wait outside.

My decision to move was rash and irresponsible. I didn't think about the consequences of not being hired. I took a huge risk moving out to Salt Lake City. An unreasonable risk, and I can only guess the universe held its breath because another decision could have possibly changed my entire career or ended the possibility of finishing my book.

He called me back in and told me I had a job. I could start immediately.

I suppose the universe let out a collective sigh. My plan concocted in the hottub was taking shape. Coaching was at first fun. Eight one-hour, 40 per week coaching sessions quickly became monotonous.

All the new business opportunities sold by the company needed merchant accounts to accept credit cards. I forget how I found Chuck, the credit card agent, but he flew out from Vancouver, Washington, to train my wife, myself, and a local hippie/computer hack I had befriended.

Things went exceptionally well for about for the first five months of 1996. Then in May, the company went bankrupt and stuck the Bank of Utah with millions in charge disputes-- chargebacks that occurred because they never delivered the merchandise paid for with their credit cards.

I was right. It was a scam all along. On top of that, things were tough at home as well. My wife had a second miscarriage; our 20-week old baby girl fell out of her uterus into my hands. I was ill-equipped emotionally to help my wife with our loss. We had no health insurance, and all of the hospital bills were absorbed into our credit card debt.

Everything was compounded by the stress of being stuck in Salt Lake without a job, no leads, and a bunch of angry merchants who had no business to run. The merchants, who lost $2000 for credit card processing software they could no longer use for their business, had paid thousands of dollars for the business opportunity and products. It was awful.

Looking back, I didn't know any better. It was the way everyone in the payment business did business. Today, just thinking about it horrifies me.

I had been submitting merchant business through Chuck's small agent office in Vancouver, Washington. So when the distressed merchandise companies died and with it all its leads, I called him and explained my predicament. He said frankly, "David, you need to get out there and begin talking to local retail merchants about accepting credit card payments. If you want to pay rent, you had better get to work."

And so, with no other choice, I began visiting local restaurants and retail businesses, which was unknown and scary because I had never done payment processing for retail companies before. After a few months of scrambling and barely making enough on equipment commissions to pay rent, Chuck made an offer to pay us a monthly salary plus commission to manage sales at his agent office in Vancouver, plus a percentage of ownership in the Agent office business.

Move to Vancouver, Washington

At the time, it was exhilarating. As I remember, we gladly left Salt Lake with a happy prospect to work with our new "visa" partners in Washington. Things seemed to go well for three months, but by August—out of the blue-—Chuck declared he was filing bankruptcy. God, what was going on? I had not checked their business financials. I know he was struggling with cash flow when our paycheck bounced, but I didn't know they had fallen so far down the rabbit hole.

Again, I was jobless. Two companies I've worked for in bankruptcies in nine months. Was this a God nod? I should just get in a truck, pack up, and drive back to Virginia Beach? But to what end? I had no job prospects there either. The Armageddon Stones manuscript and research were unfinished.

There was no money to be made there. I remember being so angry that I prayed, found a telephone book, and looked under the "accept credit cards" in the yellow pages. An 800# stood out, so I called it. Thinking it was a local number in the Portland, Vancouver area, Jack Cook answered the phone, an Agent for a card service company in Scottsdale, Arizona.

I explained to him my desperate situation. The bounced payroll check left us no money even to pay rent. Jack flew me down to Scottsdale, and after a pleasant dinner, he wrote me a $2000 check so I could pay my rent and assured me he would help me with new business leads so I could sell payment processing and make a living. He did just that.

I sold for Jack Cook for nearly two years.

In the meantime, I moved two hours north up to Olympia, Washington, because many of the merchants we set up for credit card acceptance were in Seattle. My wife had another miscarriage. The constant stress of moving around was taking its toll on all the family. The bills still piled up, nearly $70,000 in medical and credit card debt. Commission sales were not enough to keep up with the massive debt load, and after many uncomfortable weeks of indecision, we declared bankruptcy in May 1997.

With the weight around our necks gone, the credit card business grew slowly. Then one day, Dan, the owner of a local payment provider and a competitor, called me and said, "David, everywhere my reps go, we are finding your business cards. Why don't you come work for me? I responded, "Why would I do that? I am doing just fine."

He answered, "We pay monthly residuals on credit card volume. You can build a portfolio and sell it." I had never heard of such a thing. Monthly residuals based on credit card volume was a new idea. Dan explained how it worked and said, "I will pay you 50% of the residuals I make." I was taken back. I consulted others in the business, and they said it was a myth: "They won't pay you. It's a myth. No one pays residuals."

I wrestled with my decision for days. Jack had helped me when I was down and out, but this was something I couldn't ignore. It would be a considerable increase in income for my family. I had already run the numbers. I finally made the wrenching call to Jack to say I wouldn't be sending him any more business. He had been like a father to me in many ways, but I knew I had to move on.

A New Payment Model

Dan's promises turned out to be accurate. We set up a small satellite sales office over US Bank in downtown Olympia. I brought on a substantial amount of internet business, and in the midst of it all,

I helped catch my daughter Angela when she was born at St. Peters Hospital on June 7th, 1998.

The new business model attracted my Dad, who had sold real estate for the last 15 years in the Olympia area. The real estate market had dried up, and I noticed quickly he was a terrific payment salesman in the local area. Dad later ended up being our second highest producing agent for our satellite office.

By 1999, residuals topped $80,000 a year, not including commissions. Dan agreed to sell half of my portfolio for $40,000, so I could use it as a down payment to buy a house in Olympia, a remarkable feat since I had declared bankruptcy just two years before. Not only that, I learned about underwriting the risk of accepting a merchant account, as well as the ability to analyze credit card interchange and make merchant proposals. All of this came very quickly to me, as I had always been good with numbers.

During our association together, I made many contacts in the credit card industry. The internet was new then, and there were tons of internet merchants who needed to accept online payments. Cyber Source, Authorize.net, PC Charge, Verisign, Paybycheck, were a new breed of payment gateways to run secure, online payments.

We opened another satellite office in Tacoma, sharing space with Ron Ehli, who operated Paybycheck.com. Because of my association with his company, both Ron and I were invited in the winter of 1999 to Ernst & Young's second only Start to Finish project just coming out of the garage.

The company was a new payment gateway brand, and it was our job to work with nearly twenty banking experts to determine how to market and price the three owner company and bring it to the national stage. How they chose me, just an agent card agent on the street, to this day, I don't know.

The banking experts knew absolutely nothing about payment processing. Ron and I were the payment experts. The Start to Finish program required the owners to find a CEO, a process I helped with and suggested final candidates. I had recommended a banker from California, but I had listed Locke Walsh, a local businessman from Forest Hills, Illinois, a close second. The owners and the Ernst Young partners selected Locke.

Again, an irony of Fate fell before me. Locke was hired as CEO, and in turn, Locke offered me a job as the Vice-president of Sales. In return for stock and annual salary, I had to leave the credit card business—at least while I worked there. To me, it seemed like the opportunity of a lifetime. I made the quick decision and drove 29 hours straight to Chicago the following week, to join the owners and their new CEO in a newly leased 1000 square foot office in Schaumburg, Illinois.

We worked tirelessly, seven days a week, to build the technology for the gateway. New clients were difficult to come by, but they came, nonetheless. The business plan was iterated a dozen times over to raise millions to grow the company. The angel money never materialized. Locke was "difficult" is putting it mildly" most of the time, who was determined to tear down my calm demeanor.

Still, I learned more from him about business than any other person I ever knew—and loads of business stuff I would need a year later when I started my own payment company. I didn't realize it at the time, but Locke Walsh had become one of my Rice Paper Teachers. I had kept a journal of what I called "Lockism's," wise sayings about business I later lost.

My employment lasted almost exactly a year. Locke and I butted heads until finally, I said to him, "Should I leave?"

He said, "That would be preferable."

And so, with that, I left. It was February 2001. Stuck again in a city that was not my home and without a job, my wife found work as an administrative assistant for a chiropractor, and I hit the streets selling credit card processing again.

We had leased our home out in Olympia, so we had to get by in Chicago until July until we could move back into our house. It's incredible when I look back and wonder how we survived. One miracle occurred when I was asked to store a brand new ATM machine in my garage in Olympia a year before because of a default by the merchant who owned it. In the meantime, the ATM Company was acquired. After several inquiries in the shuffle, no one had any record of the $5000 ATM, so it was mine to do with as I wished. I found a merchant in Chicago who paid $5000 for it, and I had it placed there. It was precisely the money we needed to rent a U-Haul truck to move back to Olympia.

Fast Transact, Inc.

Locke must have felt a bit of remorse at accepting my resignation. He subsequently helped me start my new company, which focused primarily on credit card acceptance for internet businesses. We named our new company Fast Transact, Inc., back in our home on Indian Summer Drive.

I remember connecting our first fax and phone line out of our bedroom. I remember turning the television to watch the Twin Towers get hit on 9/11, a shocking moment I will never forget as I had worked in the World Trade Center when I lived in NYC.

Fast Transact snowballed. Within a month, we hired Mandy, a local twenty-year-old hippie, to manage customer service and terminal deployment. We were fortunate to hire some of the best people. Success isn't yours alone; it is those you surround yourself with. We built out our garage into an office, and within a year, moved into a 1000 square foot with eight employees.

By 2003, our explosive growth continued. They helped build our successful business. My thanks to so many, including Lisa, Andrea, Adriane, Shawna, and so many others. We moved into a 7,500 square foot space on Willamette Drive in Lacey, Washington, with nearly 15 employees. We had developed significant national relationships with both Go Daddy and Verisign. Before we knew it, we were building databases to manage the ever-increasing business, risk and underwriting management, service, and sales, and were quickly become a technology-focused company.

My payment gateway experience as Locke as my boss became invaluable in the future development of Fast Transact.

I convinced Locke to certify hotel credit card interchange to take advantage of the Vacation Rental business. He did, and we quickly became known for our RPM, Rental Payment Management program, a division we sold off for a nice amount of money in 2006. The cash infusion allowed us to buy an Enterprise version of Hypercom's payment gateway to control our costs.

Our jump into technology attracted competitors who wanted to buy our company. In 2007, another company offered to buy FTI, and we agreed on a cash and stock deal, but they were never able to raise money. We later had to sue them to get our company back. It was a very stressful and harrowing experience; my former friend and business partner, unknown to me, turned out to have been convicted of wire fraud.

I never thought small. In October 2008, we signed a six-year lease to occupy the entire 15,500 square foot top floor of a building that would later be called The Fast Transact building, a 20- million-dollar construction project.

Life couldn't be better. We won local awards for the fastest growing company in 2006, 2007, & 2008. Go Daddy approached us to buy part of our company. I said "no"—a decision I later regretted. What was I thinking?

We were on top of the world. But the hammer was coming. Dead Saint Bobby said it best: *There comes a time in each person's life when gold loses its luster and diamonds cease to spark; that special time, when we all start to search, and quest, and seek that hidden voice which speaks inside, yet no one hears; that particular time when all the good we do means less than a simple smile put on a strangers face by our unselfish acts of kindness.*

You can take that to the bank because money won't get you into Heaven.[29]

Financial Collapse

Our perfect little world collapsed around us one morning that same year. I heard it on the radio first. One of our merchants had, without warning, closed their offices nationwide.

---

[29] Bobby H's NDE, #776, 02.19.06, NDERF.org

I called Lisa, my controller, and CFO, and she verified the news reports. In subsequent investigations, we discovered the owners had embezzled nearly $900,000 in-class credit card deposits, transactions later charged back over the next few months. If you carry liability as we did in the payment industry, and the merchant is unable to pay for those chargebacks, guess who has to pay? We did. Fortunately, we could borrow $1,000,000 from our banking partner to cover our losses, but the $40,000 monthly payments required to pay back the four-year loan required I cut back on employees and salaries to cover the hefty installments. The financial loss rattled me to the bone.

It got worse, a lot worse.

Six months later, my controller told me something was up with our banking partner. They appeared to be having cash problems. I wondered, "How can that be?" I saw their projected EBITDA just a few months ago of $20,000,000. They were one of the largest payment processors in the industry.

Her suspicions turned out to be true. By late August 2009, our ISO partner announced they were filing Chapter 13 bankruptcy. My God. Everything we had built over the last eight years would be in jeopardy if they didn't pay us our monthly residual payment of nearly $600,000. We were a break-even company, so any interruption in our cash flow of this magnitude would be disastrous.

A scenario I never even considered or prepared for had come to pass. I couldn't sleep. My heart would not stop pounding. I prayed. I cried. And I prayed some more.

For one of the first times in my life, I was afraid.

I couldn't imagine losing my company and going out of business. In early September, we were approached by a major payment company, who offered to acquire FTI for cash and stock.

They felt confident the bankruptcy court would continue our monthly revenue payments, but the damage was done to my emotional health.

I was done.

On top of that, my marriage was in shambles. I had already separated from my now ex-wife a year earlier. I moved into my own home then courted a destructive relationship, a personal story I will not elaborate on, other than to say, it proved pivotal in my decision to build Akio Gardens.

I desperately wanted out of the payment business. I was sick of it. Literally!! I was bleeding, and in pain from ulcerative colitis, no doubt worsened by the stress of selling the company. FTI had provided financial security for many years, but it was a terrible trade-off for the havoc it created in my family and my health. So after four months of hard negotiation, we closed the sale on January 31, 2010. We stayed on as employee consultants for about a year, a typical "peeling back of the rose," unveiling company history, employee relationships, bank relationships, among other things. It was clear to me; the billion-dollar company wanted us out sooner than later.

In my company's building, I believed I had been following the breadcrumbs left by God for many years. It seemed the Yellow Leaf had been floating seamlessly downstream for many years. Perhaps I should have heard the roar of the cataract as I approached its edge.

The current was rushing over the waterfall with such tremendous force; nothing could stop the leaf from being carried with it over into the depths below. The Yellow Leaf wouldn't be destroyed in the plunge. It floated over the falls through the mist, landing gently on the river below, continuing slowly on its journey to an unknown destination.

After all attorney expenses, debt notes paid off, stock buyouts to other shareholders, we still walked away from the deal with enough money to retire on—at least that's what I thought.

13

The Fortress

Returning Wires

You must know more about this interesting story, a drama that nearly tore my life apart before the sale was consummated on January 31, 2010. On September 27, 2008, a day before my 14th Wedding Anniversary, I had a vivid dream about making a difficult decision. I was driving my old 1967 white Chevy Station Wagon as I came to a "T" at the end of a gravel road. An older, lanky gentleman with a slight beard I didn't recognize was standing on the road in front of a 10-speed bike. I came to a stop a few feet away from him and stepped out of the wagon to see what he wanted.

He looked at me with a nauseous kind of look and said, "You need to make a decision, don't you?"

I didn't respond right away.

The older man persisted, "You could turn left, and you can continue down that road. You have been there many times before. You know the way. And you will get home. You could turn to the right. It's an unknown path. He road winds through the wilderness and mountains, filled with forests, lions, tigers, and bears. It's dangerous, but it's beautiful. You can choose to turn this direction as well. It's your choice. Both roads will get you home.

I don't remember what I chose to do during the dream, but the next day, instead of choosing to take my wife out to dinner for our Anniversary, I decided to say goodbye and end our marriage. It was one of the most difficult decisions of my life, and it turned out to be one of the most dangerous, beautiful, and exciting choices of my life.

I moved out and rented a small house a few miles away to be close to my children.

The next year, I can say it was a blur. Within a few months, without going into all of the "gory" personal details, I entered a relationship that set in motion many poor decisions. However, my children never met her; it affected my children and my ex-wife's decision to move from the home we owned. It was now up to me whether I wanted to keep the house or we sell. My decision to make a "right turn" was dangerous, and over the next twelve months, I faced a "year of hell" that nearly crippled my life and my self-worth, a year which ended on December 18th, 2009, when I met Delynn, whom I married eighteen months later, August 20th, 2011.

Meeting Delynn

I began playing Texas hold 'em poker a few times a week, just to get out of the house and meet people. Sitting down for the $35 buy-in tournament, I couldn't help but stare at the beautiful, auburn-haired woman sitting across from me. I had never seen her before. During poker games, players don't usually talk, so I quietly eyed her but didn't know her name or anything about her other than she smiled a lot! It was in October 2009. I was in the middle of negotiations to sell my company, so the poker time was a welcome relief from stress.

I would later discover she had been keeping an eye on me as well. It was the night of December 18th. I sat next to her while playing poker and got her name. Delynn. It wasn't the money that brought me to the poker room. The friendship and comradery of interacting with the same players each week attracted me, especially the prospect of seeing Delynn again. I had begun playing a few more times a week, just to allow myself to see her. Asking her out for a date was uncharted waters for me, and I avoided it altogether.

It's funny that I could talk to multi-million dollar companies about business without a quibble, but asking a woman for her phone number was like jumping into cold water. I couldn't do it.

On that particular evening, lady luck wasn't with me, and by 11:00 p.m. I was out of chips. I got up to leave, and Delynn walked up to me, gave me a big smile, and asked me for my phone number, and we exchanged numbers. I gave her my number, and then I left. I got home, went to bed, and texted Delynn, "Hey, maybe we could go out for dinner sometime."

She immediately texted back, "Why not tonight?"

At the time, I was living alone in a gated apartment complex, just a mile from the casino. Of course, I jumped out of bed, got dressed, and drove five minutes back down to the casino to pick her up in my chrome-trimmed, black Ram 3500 long bed diesel truck. I had never been asked out before like this in my entire life, so when Delynn hopped into my truck, it was quite the moment for a fifty-year-old man who had never been invited out at midnight for a drink. We drove to a local bar, had a few drinks, and talked non-stop all night. We both exchanged the fact we had recently left disastrous relationships with restraining orders intact.

By the time the evening was over, we had fully informed each other of our bad and good traits, and I took her back to her car.

I asked Delynn out to dinner the next day, and after a beautiful evening out, I realized I was absolutely in love with her. I invited her to Maui to spend New Year's with me at the Grand Wailea Resort. As you can imagine, it was quite a second date. We were inseparable after that.

Delynn witnessed all the drama about the sale of my company.

The selling of Fast Transact was a major turning point in my life. I now had the funds to do anything I wanted to do or could dream of. Thinking back to my Hearthfire Lodge days with Paul Solomon and my fellow students, we had dreamed together of building a school, foremost a gardening school, teaching the greater mysteries of the universe. A school of horticulture, bonsai, vegetable and fruit gardens. Gardens with a Japanese theme and such beauty the world would take notice – a sacred space that would attract people of all faiths. I called it Akio Botanical Gardens, a name I borrowed from John Anthony West after reading a Japanese article about the root of the word "Akio," a word meaning "bright boy." I had sold my "material life" with the good intention of building a new spiritual life dedicated to the Lord.

Building Akio Botanical Gardens

The moment we moved in, I knelt down and promised God, "I will build to you a beautiful garden and home dedicated just to you." I thought I was sure this was what I was supposed to do with my life. This is my Mission. Paul, wouldn't you be proud?

I partnered with Phil Hulbert from Tsuki Nursery, Mike Z, a local heavy equipment contractor. We went to work planning and building the most extensive Japanese gardens in Washington State.

I was still quite sick from the colitis, so by May, a month after I started the garden and house remodeling project, "I thought. I will do a 40 day fast and cure myself!"

I had already done two seven day fasts in the last several months, but they had not helped my medical condition at all, so I thought perhaps a more prolonged fast would work. Eighteen days into fast, my symptoms got worse, and I had to stop. I was desperate. I didn't know what to do. I had a new life, a new partner, a new hope, a new garden being built, but I didn't have my health.

A month later, the doctors removed my appendix in an attempt to help me. I had already planned a camping trip, an appointment with my kids I had to keep. It was the first time Delynn met my kids. But removing my appendix didn't work. By the end of July, things were worse. I remember saying to God, "If you can't fix this, I want out. I can't build a school and these beautiful Gardens being so sick."

I went back to my doctor and told him I was tired of twenty-two years of the disease. I wept. He said, "David, we have tried every conventional therapy. The only option we have left is a clinical trial at Washington State University. Give Dr. Lee, who heads the program there, a call.

And so I did. By August, I was enrolled in the program, and by late October 2010, my disease was 100% in remission. My prayers were answered. The therapy worked! I was healed! Praise God!

Let's get to work and finish this garden! Let's collect the best bonsai trees, the best Japanese maple specimens, (The big ones) irrigation, stadium lights, let no expense be spared. Heck, even my contractors didn't give me a budget. Keep building! God, the place looked like Stonehenge up my driveway. David Solomon was back!

We planned, built, and planted for nearly three years. It's incredible how much money you can sink into a garden, especially a Japanese garden. Hey, why stop there? Why not buy a boat, a GTR race car, and invest in risky gold stocks? We even had an oil painting from our Belarusian friend, Iriana, of the Sistine Chapel on my ceiling; you know the one where God reaches out to touch Adam with his finger?

We had planned our wedding. Even though it was my wedding, it was one of the most beautiful weddings shared with our family and friends. Our wedding was held at the Wyndham Hotel in Virginia Beach, Virginia. August 20, 2011.

We were three years into the seven-year project when I discovered the tumor in my brain on June 13, 2013. I thought I had been fulfilling my life purpose by building these beautiful gardens with this beautiful bride.

Part III
The Withering Bosai – Removing the Wires

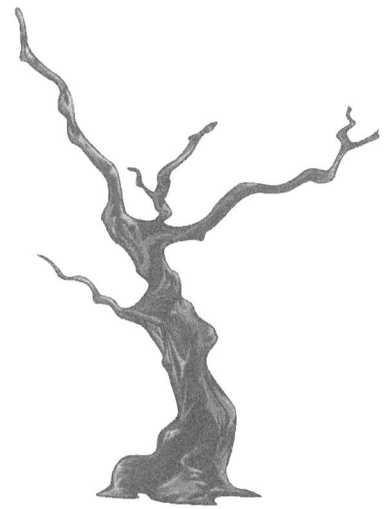

~Cancer is a real mind game. I don't want it to defeat me. Since I don't remember dying before, I have no point of reference for what it feels like to die. So the tides of my attitude ebb daily by how I feel. Mostly I try to keep my emotions in check, but from time to time, I can lose my temper in a "flash." Brain Tumor patients call it "Roid" rage or Keppra rage (taken for seizures) – a blast of emotion that lasts only minutes but is intense. It's only happened two or three times, but I beat myself up every time I "lose" it. ~**Chronicle 371**

―― 14 ――

The Tao

Cancer Communication

Daoism Taoism is a philosophical or religious tradition of Chinese origin which emphasizes living in harmony with the _Dao_ : literally: 'the Way,' The _Dao_ is a fundamental idea in most Chinese philosophical schools; in Daoism, however, it denotes the principle that is the source, pattern, and substance of everything that exists. Daoism differs from Confucianism by not emphasizing rigid rituals and social order. It is a teaching about the various disciplines for achieving "perfection" by becoming one with the unplanned rhythms of the universe called "the way" or "dao." Daoist ethics vary depending on the particular school but generally emphasize we wei (action without intention), "naturalness," simplicity, spontaneity, and the three treasures: compassion, frugality, and humility. 慈 "compassion," 儉 "frugality," and 不敢為天下先 "humility."

Virginia Beach, VA
My friend called me out of the blue in early September 2006. We had not spoken to one another since our mutual teacher and friend, Paul Solomon, who had died in March 1994. I lived in Washington State, near Olympia, the state capital, since then, and had slowly lost contact with many of my former co-students and East Coast friends.

When he called me on that September day 2006, he told me he had terminal brain cancer. He didn't say what kind of brain cancer it was or how long he had to live. He had no insurance, but the local hospital donated funds for surgery to remove or "resect" the small, marble-sized brain tumor, which had grown near the base of his brain.

At the time, I didn't know anything at all about brain cancer, its voracious, aggressive type, or how long he had to live. I just knew in my gut that he needed to get his house in order. And I promptly told him so. Though I was concerned, he seemed so optimistic he would beat his cancer that failure was just not an option for him.

He had decided to go to Mexico for a natural alternative treatment. Time slipped by, and I assumed that the treatment worked. Three months later, I got a call that he was not expected to live much longer.

My first thought was, "Why didn't anyone notify me sooner? Why didn't I check on him?"

At the time, I was CEO of my own company and was impossibly busy. Yet I felt I needed to be there. I made arrangements with my employees and family to run things, got on a plane, and headed for Virginia Beach.

When I arrived, I didn't know what to expect. I had no details about the situation. The shock of seeing him lay prostrate on a hospital bed made me realize I had never actually sat with anyone who may die in my presence. He was only 55. For some reason, the death of friends and family happened when I was not around. It always was someone else's experience, something you hear about in the news or read in a book.

My first exposure to death was the tragic accident of my mother's second husband, Jack, who was killed in a freak accident in October 1984 while trimming a large tree in his friend's back yard. A branch had split unexpectedly in two, falling and killing him instantly.

I had been ordained by the Fellowship of the Inner Light, October 16, 1983, but I had spent most of my time traveling and assisting with Teaching and Healing ministries. I never pastored a church or performed a funeral. I just didn't run into dead and dying people.

When Jack died, I was a young pastor, only 25 years old. Mom asked me to perform his memorial service, which was no small event since he had been an active military. Five-hundred people came to the funeral, accompanied, of course, by an American Flag over the casket, Flag folding, handover of the flag to Mom, and a 21-gun salute.

All these memories flooded in as I sat down next to my friend's bed. To my surprise, he lifted his right hand, *the only part of his body he could still move*, to acknowledge me, and said, "David, I am glad you could make it," his voice clear as a bell.

He was only ten days away from passing over.

He had no use of any of his motor functions, except for his right foot and right hand. His eyes were closed, and he could lie comfortably on his left side. He was conscious, able to talk, and was still sipping broth and drinking water. It had only been five months since diagnosis.

Hospice managed his care, providing his family and friends with morphine drops for headaches and suppositories for nausea. He was, in fact, very comfortable most of the time. Ever since I knew him, he was a natural supplement, a workout kind of guy, and one of the healthiest people I knew. He looked 45, not 55, his hair still Italian jet black, his body in perfect physical form from daily exercise. He did not look like a man who was dying.

In the last several days before his death, I noticed many of us wondered when he would die. I guess it's just a natural thing to think about. The hospice nurse came around dinnertime every day and checked his vitals. She told us he could hang on for several more days because he was so healthy

Late one night, when the family was asleep, I had my chance to spend time with him. It was just five days before he passed away. Holding his hand, I told him, "You know, the doctors believe you will die within just a few days. Do you realize this?" He squeezed my hand, and weakly replied, "Really?"

I whispered, "Yes." He nodded and said, "Wow, I didn't know."

He was drifting in and out of consciousness, but I continued gently talking with the man I considered my best friend and got the courage up to ask him a tough question. "What does it feel like...knowing you are going to die soon?"

A few seconds passed, then he said, "Well, it's like I am standing on a cliff, and I can only see darkness below. I don't know what is down there. I'm a little afraid because it is unknown, but on the one hand, I am a little excited too. I feel like something awesome is about to happen." He then drifted back to sleep.

The following day, I could see he was drifting between this world and the Afterlife. He began talking to those we could not see. He lifted his hand and motioned to me, "Paul Solomon is here. He says he loves you. "It's so very beautiful here. So many colors...."

Another day passed. I had the "night watch" and was sitting alone with him around 4:00 a.m., when he quietly blurted out, "David, I think this is it. I'm going to pass now."

Yikes! I woke everybody up. Friends rushed over to be by his side. By 6:00 a.m., he let out a sigh and smiled,

"Well, I guess that was a trial run."

Everyone cracked up and, after a bit, went back to bed or back home.

Another day went by, and without warning, he stopped speaking, drinking, and drifted off into a coma. Two days later, he began hyperventilating like a fish out of water. It went on for about an hour. I held his left hand and a church friend (who strangely died of cancer a year later) held his right hand. Without thinking, like calming a baby to sleep, I suddenly leaned over and whispered in his ear, "Shhhhhhhh. It's okay."

He immediately stopped breathing, and an electric shock passed through my arm and body. He took one last breath, and at that moment, he let go of his body, stepped off the cliff, and dove into the unknown. Even though he could not communicate with me verbally, I am quite sure he beamed "goodbye, my friend," as his spirit departed this life for the next.

The honest truth is, as my friend died, I thought to myself, "Geeze, that's not a bad way to go. It's not violent. Not too painful. I would have time to say goodbye to my family. Sure, why not? That's the way I'd like to die."

~Cancer is a real mind game. I don't want it to defeat me. Since I don't remember dying before, I have no point of reference for what dying feels like. So the tides of my attitude ebb daily by how I feel. Mostly I try to keep my emotions in check, but from time to time, I can lose my temper in a "flash." Brain Tumor patients call it "Roid" rage or Keppra rage (taken for seizures) – a blast of emotion that lasts only minutes but is intense. It's only happened two or three times, but I beat myself up every time I "lose" it. ~**Chronicle 371**

~Sunday, October 4th, 2014 – Meeting Paul Michels and John Forte. Delynn had met Paul and John at Chops, our local restaurant, which is below our apartment. We went there regularly, but Delynn went more often. She would sometimes go to edit some of the books or just to decompress after a long day. When I became aware that Paul and John were in the filming industry, I asked if they had known my friend who had died of GBM in 2007. Their jaws dropped. In an excited voice, John said, "You know him?" The same one who acted for Coastal Video during the 1990s? It's such a small world, after all, even in Virginia Beach, with a population of 1 million.

~Monday, October 5th: Writing my ass off. Finished Chapter 8: Rice Paper Teachers; Chapter 9: The Book of Life; and Chapter 12: We Die in Character. Many of the chapters are 80% done. I just need commentary, edits, and conclusions.

~October 7th, 2014 – Dream of crossing a river holding on to a pole attached to a robe spanning the river. Observed a trout swimming below the thin ice and an orange (tropical) ice and tropical mix like my original near-death dream in 2013 when I saw Grandma Miller. ~October 8th, 2014 – Dream of asking Grace de Rond to help ghostwrite and finish the DSC.

~John Anthony West speaking at the ARE this weekend. I wanted to give him the first 13 chapters. John and Celesta came to visit.

~October 24, 2014 – Dream of a swimming pool in the basement. 55-degree water. That's is very, very cold, but it felt warm. Just fine. Of course, the number that stands out is '55'. 55 years old. My 56th birthday is January 23, 2015....three months from now. And the water feels warm. It feels "fine." Hmmm...tempting, inviting.

~October 29, 2014 – Dream - I am in the "President's Mansion." Paul Solomon and Bicameral Mind- One Mind- Shekinah – Can't teach a student how to do this. It depends on the student. A moment of prayer – the miraculous. A Coal of fire from off the altar. Touch it to your lips.... that your heart may be pure....that you may become a spokesman for Christ.

~October 30, 2014 - Dream- pebbles just under the water leading towards bridge crossing river. 6 San Souci relaxed summer chairs freshly painted blue and grey. The pebbles made me look like I was walking on water. (another death symbol- bridge & river).

~October 31, 2014 - Dream- Mr. Takanohashi- Nebari – slicing bread/cutting the bread in half. Bread represents book-spiritual teaching. Give us this day, our daily bread...And then cutting the book in half. I was only a week away from sending the Chronicles' rough draft to John Anthony West for editing when Mr. Takanohashi, my deceased bonsai teacher, appeared in a dream. Pointing at an old azalea trunk and its thick, exposed roots and gruffly said *Nebari!*. Nebari is a Japanese word that means *root, specifically the visible spread of roots above the growing medium at the base of a bonsai*. When I studied with Mr. Takanohashi in Japan in the late 1980s (*a story I expand in Book III; The Galileo code*), he always said *Nebari*, with such great passion. It was the second time he had visited me during an ADC dream, the last time only a few months before. He had died in the late 1990s, but I had not seen him since 1989. I said to him in the dream, "You're alive!" He just grinned at me, and then the dream was over.

Journal Entries Grappling with GBM

~Chemo treatments allow me to purchase time. So far, on the surface, this appears to be true. At some point in the next several months, it will be fewer drugs and more God blessing me with time.

Family drama about the purchase of the cars my children needed and with their mother. Sometimes, it's easier to write about the Dead Saints' stories than deal with family issues. I've got to work handler to make things better. When it comes to family, sometimes communication; the Zen Koan applies: You do not know what you do not do. ~**Chronicle 427**

~It's the 377th day since my tumor discovery. How do I feel now, as compared to a few months back in April, March, February, or January, for that matter? Not really any different. The wonkiness and disorientation are the same. My attitude is just a bit better. I have iterated the outline so often that I feel like I am lost in a groundhog writing time loop. I've got to pick one and just stick with it. I even had a dream that I was locked out of the Editor's office. ~**Chronicle 377**

~Across the threshold of the veil, lies another world. It is a realm of imagination that so thoroughly impresses a Dead Saint's mind they know their encounter with the Afterlife was more than an illusion. It is a real experience. Carol Zeliski asks a great question in *Life in the World to Come*: 'Do NDEs create undo "saccharine" optimism about the Afterlife?' I don't think so. A friend of mine said that I seemed a little too excited about dying. Perhaps, I need to cool down my "saccharine" optimism about crossing over. I guess the Afterlife evidence I have discovered gives more meaning to life.[30] ~**Chronicle 389**

~Another 45-minute boring MRI at Hampton VA center. The loud racket of the MRI machine requires earplugs. But it does nothing to quiet the mind. I wondered, 'How was I going to heal myself of this tumor? Will I have to die and have a near-death supernatural instantaneous healing moment? Or was I going to tell God, 'Hey, I am not ready to die yet?'~ **Chronicle 411**

---

[30] *Carol Zeliski Life in the World to Come.*

~I looked at the four gelatin Temodar pills in my palm. After twelve months and sixty chemo treatments, I arrived at my last month of chemical punishment. Just sixteen more pills to take over the next four days. I should be excited, but I am not. Delynn asked me if I wanted to go downstairs and have a drink with her friends. I told her, 'No. You go ahead. I'm not feeling up to it. It's okay.'

I was lying.

After she left, I looked at the wet laundry in front of the washer, picked up a colored damp towel, and threw it hard against the wall. God, I hate this. I'm sick of feeling drugged. I'm sick of feeling tired. I'm sick of being sick. I want to go down and have a drink with my wife and her friends, but I simply don't feel like it. The neuro-oncologist says the Temodar will take 60-90 days to get out of my blood. So perhaps by December, I will begin to feel better? She wants me off the Dex too. More crap to deal with. ~**Chronicle 445**

~As a grapple with my disease, I feel I have learned much. I guess my Life Review will bear witness if I have gained a bit of wisdom here and there. I have observed in others and myself that only a handful change bad habits and ineffective ways of living—even when we are aware of them. ~**Chronicle 583**

~I pulled my old telescope parts box out of the proverbial procrastination mothballs. I thought I remembered I had ground the mirror more. I'm not even close to a ground mirror with an F8/64- inch focal length. Finishing the project requires a few weeks of grinding (and the energy to stand up doing it) polishing, a $100 coating of aluminum, an 8-inch cardboard tube, and a stand. I can buy the same 8-inch telescope on e-Bay for $300. It's a nice fantasy to finish grinding the mirror...but it probably won't happen. Finishing the book comes first. ~**Chronicle 780**

~Angela called. She cried and said she misses me and wants to come home. She says she would be happier in Virginia. Angela feels she is choosing happiness over her college future. Of course, her future is what she makes of it. I told Delynn it would be a miracle if she came home to Virginia. Angela is undecided, so I wait. Bad cold. In bed. I have to be careful of pneumonia. ~**Chronicle 789**

~Unknown to me, my sister Terri had been talking with Angela all week by phone. When Angela called me and said, "she was coming home" to Virginia, I knew right then Terri had helped her make an impossible decision, leave her mother in Washington, and finish her senior year at Cox High School. Angela wants a Prom. She wants a formal High School. She followed her heart. She wants to be with me because the next year will most likely my last. ~**Chronicle 804**

DREAM: Jesus and I were staring at each other. He was only an arms-length away. I could only see his face. Jesus no longer wore a crown of thorns. Where sharp thorns had pierced his forehead and scalp, BB-sized puncture wounds filled with coagulated bright red blood remained. His long hair was matted with blood. His beard was gone, revealing deep wounds from 39 lashes he received before the crucifixion. The long scars on his face were also filled with blood. Jesus appeared bruised and beaten. He looked rough. It was as if Jesus wanted me to know what He looked like after rising from the dead, with his crown of thorns removed, his face shaven, revealing the full extent of his injuries. I believe Jesus wanted me to know how much he suffered—for me. I then woke up. ~**Chronicle 934** 1.2.16

~Angela texted to get help to pay for half her gorgeous Prom Dress last night. Ordered her dress on my 57th Birthday-Jan 23, 2016. Getting closer to reaching day 1103 and Angela's School graduation!!!
~**Chronicle 955**

―――― 15 ――――

The Termination

Death Wires

~Cancer is like a near-death experience without the associated Death Elements of dying. And like an NDE, it profoundly affected my soul. When I meet someone and find out about my cancer, I can see that it sometimes makes them uncomfortable—a few resort to looking down at the floor or losing eye contact with me. So I have learned not to disclose, if possible, my condition. ~**Chronicle 391**

Dying Decisions: Compensating Forces During Terminal Illness
When someone approaches their appointed time, it appears there are two sets of fates that come into play, compensating forces of free will and faith that occur during terminal illness or old age. I believe this is precisely the case in my predicament. But how much can I adjust or change that destiny, even if it is pre-ordained?

According to Dion Fortune, "The power of will and faith of a dying person may be sufficient delay death, but usually, within several months, Fate will run its course until death ensues. If free will or faith interrupts death, we then may sign a new lease on life. When that happens, according to some mystics, there is little likelihood of death until the planets have once again moved into a fatal position."[31]

Do we have free will, or is it an illusion? Depending on who you read, yes and no. Is it ultimately a theology of giving up your free will to follow God's will? According to the Dead Saints, we mustn't give up our free will. We must choose between right and wrong, good and evil.

---

[31] Dion Fortune, Through the Gates of Death

But the lesson is not just about making choices. The task is to make free will choices that serve God's divine plan.

Even Jesus faced a momentous decision in the Garden of Gethsemane. He had to choose to allow himself to be brutally crucified. The legends describe Christ "sweat blood" over his decision to follow his Father's Will. He made a choice not to run away from his destiny—and more importantly, he did not give up his ability to decide. Christ chooses to do what He came here to do and what his Father in Heaven wanted Him to do.

It is a choice. The right thing to do is written within our hearts. So what does it mean? It is a paradox; to have the free will to choose "rightly" and follow God's will. How do we know what God's will is? How do we reconcile this typical wrangling within the soul?

Here's an analogy about following God's will that I think makes sense. When you drive an automobile, it won't drive itself. You must press the gas and hold onto the steering wheel–analogous to your requirement to make life decisions. God won't do this for you. However, the route you take, your destination is up to you. Your destination is God's Divine Will.

The ultimate question is, "How do I know God's will?" How do you know which way to turn when you reach a fork in the road? How do you choose?

Driving is usually an unconscious act because you go the same route to work or back home again every day. Sometimes you alter your driving route to perform an errand or pick up groceries. You make minor decisions every day concerning your driving route to home or work, but you always know your destination. You wouldn't just take off to a South Pacific island because you just decided to do so. If you have responsibilities to family or friends or work, you will tell them if you made such a decision.

If it seems complicated, if it looks like you are fighting against the current, you can bet your decision to do so is not in your best interest or God's best interest.

I learned this principle from T'ai Chi. If you apply too much force, usually something will break. So whether in driving or watching a yellow leaf flow downriver, it naturally occurs, without using too much force that generally determines the right decision.

Making a free will choice is one of the most misunderstood lessons presented by Earth University. It is a lesson we should pay close attention to.

~The key to knowing God's will, His preferred path, is understanding resistance. In electronics, a resistor integrated into a circuit board restricts the flow of electricity. If the resister is not there, the flow of electricity moves through a wire unimpeded. This "unimpeded" flow is God's preferred path. David, what do you mean? I think we intuitively understand when life is happily moving along, and everything is "magically" falling into place. I believe this means we are walking on God's preferred path. However, when I make free-will decisions that cause problems in my life, it will feel like resistance—not the preferred path.

I have used the analogy of a yellow leaf floating downstream. The yellow leaf will float happily along with the current but will encounter boulders, logs, and rapids that may impede its journey downriver. These obstacles are the Earth University tests. Have you learned your lessons? If you have, you won't run into the same rock again. Next time, it will be different. The key is how to navigate around the rock by understanding the resistance of the rock. There is a preferred path along God's river of life.

Principle: Water wears away the stone

If I encounter resistance, it means I have encountered a decision, a choice, to bring balance—to overcome it—by force, or crushing it by applying the power of softness—LOVE. Thus the ancient T'ai Chi philosophy, "Water wears away the stone," applies. How often have I used force, causing breakage in physical objects, family communications, and relationships?

If I run into resistance, take it as God's breadcrumb. It means I need to change the direction I am headed. Sometimes the opposition comes from others. What does it mean? If it is my resistance, my ego, I need to stop for a moment and look for the truth. Is it me? If so, and I want to balance the resistance, I need to let go of my OPINIONS. If the resistance is in others, then God's breadcrumb may be telling me to work out the relationship. If not, then move on. Our growth comes from solving these resistances. They appear as problems, but the truth lies in making a non-placating decision that causes a release of resistance and the re-establishment of balance. ~**Chronicle 986 – February 24, 2016**

~Sitting placidly on my ocean facing balcony in Virginia Beach. My two bonsai, the 150-year-old Western Juniper and 90-year-old rhododendron stand watch like pillars of Jachin and Boaz on either side of me, while Venus twinkles brightly in the morning dawn, waiting for the golden sun to break through the ripples of a gentle sea -- pondering the meaning of the Old Testament statements; walking before God, walking with God, and walking after God.

To walk is to live; as to walk in the law, to walk in the statutes, and to walk in the truth. It is a term used in Genesis referring to Enoch and Noah 6:9, as "a just man, perfect in his generations, [who] walked with God." It is a term applicable to each of us today not just in Old Testament times. What happens when we walk with someone?

Imagine you and a close friend are enjoying a walk through the forest side by side. You talk, laugh, listen, and share your hearts. Your attention is focused on this person to the exclusion of almost everything else. You seem to know their thoughts, and they know yours. You are in harmony. I believe, walking with God is like that. In Genesis 17:1, we read, "I am Almighty God; walk before Me and be blameless" When we live before God, it is a movement toward holiness --nothing to hide- to have a clear conscience. How do you begin walking in holiness? Tell ourselves the truth. ~ **Chronicle 369**

A few days earlier:

~Delynn's daughter Leah, got a distressed call from her husband in Afghanistan. Two soldiers in his platoon in Afghanistan were killed in a UN friendly fire incident because of bad targeting intelligence. In his grief, he punched a cement wall in anger and shattered his hand. Due to the injury which required surgery, he had to report back to Fort Carson in Colorado.

Leah didn't know whether to cry for Jason's loss or be overwhelmed with joy at his return safely home from his 4th tour of Afghanistan – alive. ~**Chronicle 367**

Can the stars predict our death?

Some believe that the stars can predict the time of death with great accuracy. According to Dion Fortune, "There are tides of death on every soul's horoscope, tides on which the soul may slip across the great harbor into the vast beyond." [32]

I got a Hindu dose predictive horoscopes when a Vedic Astrologer visited me in July 2015. He heard about my cancer and asked a friend from our church to bring him over to my house to see.

---

[32] Dion Fortune, Through the Gates of Death

To make conversation, as neither of us had met before, I asked him on a hunch to read my unedited chapter on *Jesus, Planetary Headmaster*. He didn't put it down until he had read all of it. His face had a look of surprise—an OMG look. He was raised Catholic, and later, he fell in love with Hindu theology because it seemed so similar to Christianity.

He said, "I've read a lot of things about Jesus written by Christian and Hindu theologians, but after reading your chapter, I understand Jesus better now than ever before. Things I hadn't put together now make perfect sense."

We talked a bit about his life as a Judge, and then he mentioned the tragic death of his teenage daughter some twenty-years earlier in a deadly auto accident. He said, "The emotional trauma of her death changed my life. I needed to find answers as to "why it happened." Was it meant to be? He spent years learning Vedic Astrology and eventually ran a chart on my daughter's date of death. It was absolutely clear. The chart indicated she was supposed to die on that very day as if the auto accident was Fated to happen.

It made me think. Could you do a chart like that for me? Like an experiment? Before admonishing me on scripture—not to seek astrologers' advice—remember this was not advice, but a science experiment! Remember, the wise men who adored Christ as a child was called Magios, a Greek word meaning, *Oriental Astrologers.*

He said: "I've never done that before. Not because I can't do it, but I believe most people can't handle such foreknowledge."

I persisted. "But will you do it?" He drummed his fingers on the table.

"Vedic Horoscopes are very, very accurate. The chart will predict a time when there is a likelihood you will die. Some death 'windows' are absolute and set in stone. Some death windows are "opportunities" where we might die, but may not because we choose to continue our mission on Earth."

"I will go home and think about it. Can we meet tomorrow before I leave?"

"Of course." The meeting was set.

He came back the next day at 1:00 p.m. on the dot. You may think it a dreadful thing on my part, but I just don't see it that way. I wanted to know "when" because I believe it's important, I know. Studies show that 96% of people don't want to know when they will die. I know I was putting him on the spot, but he didn't flinch at all.

"David, most people couldn't handle knowing when they will die, but after praying about it, I know you can. At first, I wasn't going to tell anyone and keep it just between him and me, but when he pulled out the chart, I thought I should let Delynn know about the "Death window" as well. I didn't want her reading about the prediction in my Chronicle notes after the fact. I could hear it now. Really? And you didn't think I could handle it?" Yep. Got to keep the wife happy.

He went through the same process of advancing my Natal (birth) Chart, Indian Vedic style, to a period in the future that would indicate when I might die.

His conclusion: my "death window" was between January 23, 2016 (my 57th birthday), and March 27, 2016. That's when I "might" die.

He didn't know about my prayer to live to see my daughter's graduation on June 18th, 2016. I felt like I could handle the truth, but the prediction was ninety days short of my goal. I suddenly felt like the hero in the movie, *the Martian*, who would die on Mars because he ran out of food a few weeks short of being rescued.

I needed to find a way to reach June 18, 2016. I need to find a way to survive until the 1101st day—the number of days between June 13, 2013, and June 18th, 2016. Angela's High School Graduation.

To break the "death window" barrier, I needed at least a short term life extension from God. Complete healing would be ideal, but a little more time to reach my goals would do. There is Biblical precedence for God extending life. In 2 Kings, 20:5-7, King Hezekiah was terminally ill. He was dying and prayed fervently to live. Scripture says God added fifteen years to his life: *"Return and say to Hezekiah, the leader of My people, 'Thus says the LORD, the God of your father David, "I have heard your prayer, I have seen your tears; behold, I will heal you. On the third day, you shall go up to the house of the LORD. "I will add fifteen years to your life, and I will deliver you and this city from the hand of the king of Assyria; I will defend this city for My own sake and My servant David's sake." Then Isaiah said, "Take a cake of figs." And they took and laid it on the boil, and he recovered...."*

God, are you listening?

The question yet languishes. "Do we have the right to choose our time of death?"

On July 15, 2013, just a few weeks after my GBM diagnosis, I had a Dream of Death, symbolically a dream of my future death, where I was offered a choice terminate my life: I was in the ocean surf in Kauai, Hawaii. I was hit by a massive wave and pushed hard towards the shoreline. I knew the shoreline represented Heaven. I heard someone yell from behind me that "three more waves are coming." Then, the dream shifts to a scene in a Prison. I am standing behind a woman with short, dark hair who has been sentenced to death. There is a one-inch plastic tube coming out of the left side of her skull where my tumor was supposed to be. Standing directly behind her, I am the executioner. She is sentenced to a "mercy" death by poison.

I was in charge of releasing the poison. I asked her if she were ready to receive the poison.

She said, "Yes." I released the poison, and she died instantly.

Perhaps, I will get an extra drip or two of morphine during hospice to help things along. Who knows? I don't plan to leave this life prematurely out of the fear of pain.

~Talked to Gabe, a business associate, who knew of my battle with cancer and writing of my book. We were talking about his mother, who was in a coma. I suggested he speak to her even while she was in a coma. I assured Gabe she could hear him. He did just that, and the next day she came out of her coma and called her family to the hospital. Kind of freaked everybody out. Thank you, God! ~**Chronicle 518**

"Our Time" is it Divinely Appointed?

Sometimes our date and time of death appear to be a Divine appointment. On July 4, 1826, Adams, the second president, and Jefferson, the third president, both died, exactly 50 years after adopting the Declaration of Independence. The country took it as a sign of American divinity. But there is no proof to the long-told story that Adams at 90, dying, uttered, "Jefferson survives," which was said to be especially poignant, as Jefferson had died just hours before at the age of 82, without Adams knowing it. Was Adams mistaken, or did Jefferson's spirit appear to Adams just before his death? Was it a divine coincidence, or did God plan their deaths before they were born?

Emanuel Swedenborg suffered a stroke just before Christmas in 1771 and was partially paralyzed and confined to bed. His health improved somewhat, but he died on March 29, 1772. In February, he wrote a letter to John Wesley, the founder of Methodism, saying he (Swedenborg) had been told in an after-death communication that he would die on March 29, 1772. (Wesley later read and commented extensively on Swedenborg's work.)

Swedenborg's landlord's servant girl, Elizabeth Reynolds, also said Swedenborg had predicted this date and that Swedenborg was as happy about it as if he was "going on holiday or to some merrymaking.)[33]

Are We Given Exit Points?

There may be more than one period in our life where the Angel of Death has passed.

When I look back over my life, I remember three distinct possibilities to have been killed. I do not know if it was just an accident that passed by me, or whether, on some level, I chose to remain on Earth and carry out my mission:

Age 7: Stuck a screwdriver into a Christmas light set. Electric shock blue up the screwdriver. I was not electrocuted. The same year, our house caught on fire...but we all survived.

Age 16: Choking game. NDE.

Age 18: Installing a 220v dryer with my Father. We had to work outside to bring the 220v line from the circuit breaker into the house. Dad improperly bent the pipe the wire was threaded through, exposing the copper wire against the galvanized steel pipe. When I touched the metal with a screwdriver, the 220v current blew up the screwdriver in a bright electric blue flash. If either my father or I had handled that pipe, we most likely would have been electrocuted since we were grounded to the dirt outside.

I am sure that if you are at least 55, you can recall at least two or three incidents where you could have died and taken the opportunity to leave this life but didn't.

---

[33] Wikipedia: Emanuel Swedenborg, *"Documents concerning the life and character of Emanuel Swedenborg"*. Johann Friedrich Immanuel Tafel - Google Books. Books.google.com. Retrieved 2012-08-16.

What about Suicide? Is it wrong? The authors DO NOT ENDORSE, ENCOURAGE OR ADVOCATE FOR SUICIDE IN ANY WAY, SHAPE OR FORM! If you are feeling suicidal, please know help is available. Though you may feel alone, YOU ARE NOT ALONE! If you are in crisis, call 911 IMMEDIATELY, or contact the Suicide Crisis Hotline in your state or country. Suicide Lifeline: Call 1-800-273 TALK (8255).

Are there mitigating circumstances that make one suicide right and other suicides wrong?

Christian orthodox doctrine considers suicide—all suicides—a "grave" or severe sin. Until very recently, victims of suicide were not even buried in church cemeteries. In 1997, The Catholic church published[34] a less critical view of suicide and indicated that the person who committed suicide may not always be entirely right in their mind; and thus not one-hundred-percent morally culpable: *"Grave psychological disturbances, anguish, or grave fear of hardship, suffering, or torture can diminish the responsibility of the one committing suicide."* The Catholic Church "Prays for those who have committed suicide, knowing that Christ shall judge the deceased fairly and justly."

According to the World Health Organization (WHO) in 1999, suicide is among the top ten causes of death for all age groups in North America and most northern and western European countries; it represents 1 to 2 percent of total mortality.

Suicide: Brave, Cowardly, Honorable?

When we take a closer look at suicide, there are many different situations where one suicide may differ from other suicide. Is there a time when suicide is honorable?

---

[34] *Catechism of the Catholic Church*

In Japan, the "Banzai charge" was considered one method of *Gyokusai* "jade shards" —honorable suicide before being captured by the enemy.

The origin of such beliefs was the Classical Chinese text in the 7th century called *Book of Northern Qi*, which states, "A man would rather be a shattered jade than be a complete roof tile."

Since the Sengoku period in Japan, samurai followed the code called *bushido*, defining behaviors loyal and honorable. Among the rules, there existed "honor" that was later used by Japanese military governments. Impressed with how samurai were trained to commit suicide when a great humiliation was about to befall them, the government educated troops that it was a greater humiliation to surrender to the enemy than to die. The suicide of Saigo Takamori, the leader of old samurai during the Meiji Restoration, also inspired the nation to idealize and romanticize death in battle and to consider suicide an honorable final action.

Suicide, whether romanticized by the Japanese doctrine of Bushido, or life-ending swallowing of the "poison pill" as "honorable deaths" are not typical. In most cases, it is not fear that drives their last act of free will to end their lives. Suicide, for them, becomes a statement of courage, purpose, and belief in the Afterlife.

Most suicides, however, are not born of well-thought-out endings. Most are rash acts born of desperation to escape the mental and the emotional agony of witnessing or experiencing pain. And it is this type of suicide, the deliberate aborting of their Earth University Mission.

I believe there is a" root cause" to think that leaving through suicide is a mistake. I also think those who commit rash acts of suicide do not understand the repercussions of their choice to leave Earth University "early." In all near-death experience cases I have read and researched, God responds to suicides in a loving, non-condemning manner.

However, there are repercussions to acts of rash suicide. Lisa, only 13- years-old, discovers that her decision to commit suicide and drown herself was pushing things in a way that was like an intentional "act of disobedience:"

Lisa: *With this intention [to die] I had I felt God showed me that if I did decide to go against what I knew He wanted for me at that time (which was to live) that I would be causing great disobedience in my life. I could FEEL this friction of disobedience—that I was pushing things.' This felt very uncomfortable so I decided then to get up out of the water mainly for that reason alone even though I also knew I didn't want my mother to suffer any grief over me. I realized that this was a supernatural experience I was permitted as a type of lesson about suicide's repercussions.*[35]

Suicide repercussions when it's "not your time"

It's a cause/effect universe. Nicole discovers when it is not your "time to go" that there are repercussions to suicide: *This wasn't my first suicide attempt, yet I can promise you, this most definitely will be my last. A month ago, I decided to end my own life, basically by downing sleeping pills, my other medications, and Gin, a side order of Ginseng tea. No kidding. I laid back in my bed, literally, and played the CD, A Rush of Blood to the Head, by Coldplay all night long.*

---

[35] Lisa A's NDE, #1619, 03.01.11, NDERF.org

I began to at first, sleep like a log, then somewhere during that night, I awoke, frightened. I felt my entire body shut down, literally, beginning with my mind. Each compartment was as if they were rooms and persons were turning out the lights, to leave for the night, or practically forever, and it scared me so much so, I remember standing up, kicking my legs...honestly not wanting to believe the drowsy effect taking me over.

I was so frightened, not even of dying. Still, because I just realized, my grandmother would open the door of my bedroom, and see me lying cold and dank in my bed, with this velvet light blaring over me...my body, frozen, my limbs solid, and my eyes literally open staring up at the ceiling. I realized she would see me this way.

So frighteningly, I began to push myself, to fight the haze, to fight against the tiredness I was feeling... to fight against death.

I kept saying, 'No, this isn't happening! I won't die, can't be dying! If I am talking, my eyes are open, here I am. People like me don't die. I can't let her see me lying in bed, cold, and sick. With my eyes open, please don't let me die, not like this.'

[Then] either a Seraphim or God himself, flew right over my sleeping body (my spirit returned to my body, and waited to be collected by angels) and said, in the most loving of voice. "I can't take you now honey, I'm sorry." I also heard the same voice *God* who said, "I'm sorry doll, but sometimes when people attempt suicide, and it's not their time to go, they end up in situations just to pass that time away, until it's time for that lifetime to end. And sometimes they end up in situations such as this. This is what happens." The voice was so soothing, so loving, I knew this was a time to learn.

It concluded with a kind, but quite realistic, "You will wake up." You will be in one hundred percent shape. Your mind will be 100% healthy as it always was, but when this is over, you will wake up *very* sick. Perhaps this will discourage you from future tries. Please, I am begging, your life will be beautiful, I promise you. You have nothing to worry about, you won't be homeless in the street (I was always worried that I wouldn't graduate high school or be able to take care of myself) this is a promise, from me to you. Please trust in me. I promise to never let you fall.'

After this, I remember waking up in full sound mind as promised, and as promised I was sick for three days straight, vomiting everything up (this was the body's defense to make sure I wouldn't ingest anything harmful, I know this now), but after those three days, I healed up back to the normal me.[36]

Never give up!

There is a hilarious scene in the movie *Galaxy Quest*, when the captain keeps saying over and over, "Never give up!" A simple statement I often have to keep telling myself.

Richard, who drowned himself in a suicide attempt in 2002, was not judged, but told basically to never give up. He had work to do: *That is when I remember my body falling away. I didn't leave my body it just fell away and I had the feeling I had lost a friend. It was a terrible feeling of loss and I realized I was dead. But I'm still aware! I was very aware. I remember thinking, 'I should be seeing a tunnel and some light,' but I was more like thought in space, completely alone in nothingness. So I waited and waited.*

---

[36] Nicoles' NDE, #330, 11.04.03, NDERF.org

Then the reality of what I'd just done hit me, 'I am going to be here in this place forever! This abyss! What have I done?' The fear was off the charts. We are not supposed to take our own life. I was fully aware of what I had done and the thought of being alone in that nothing forever was unbearable but what could I do? It was too late.

Suddenly in the void, I heard a voice. A male voice and He said, 'It's o.k. It's all right. It's all good.' I went from total terror to total peace and acceptance of my life and responsibility. I was no longer worried about Heaven or hell or my death. This voice accepted me and did not judge me.

I, in a way, had judged myself and clearly had an instant understanding of my life, and how important it is to play our lives out to the end regardless of how hard it is.[37]

Linda says we would stay alive as long as we can: *Death, even the meanest, cruelest and horrendous path we take prior to the moment of death, has purpose. The death of one can save many. (This has many multiple meanings that I was shown) Death of any kind is not a punishment. Death is never a punishment. Death is a shutting of the eyes and walking over into life again. Death is going home to the beginning. Death IS the beginning not the end. God does not cause our deaths, we accept death. We accepted it a long, long time ago when we were first created as Spiritual beings. God acknowledges that we have chosen to leave this life.*

It is rare when God does not allow us to die at the time of our choosing. We have the gift (or the curse) of freewill and that does not change when we make the decision to die. It is our job to stay alive as long as we can. I think that on a spiritual level and I had fought for that life.[38]

---

[37] Richard L's NDE, #1472, 01.13.08, NDERF.org
[38] Linda B's NDE #455, 08.11.04, NDERF.org

My wife, Delynn, lost two young brothers to suicide. Their choices caused great pain within her family. One brother returned to visit her in a vivid dream 32 years after his suicide. The dream was so real; it was like reliving a memory. He communicated to her that he was "okay."

Fight with everything you are, and at that moment where your life may hang in the balance, you will find out what you thought was impossible is now possible.

The Appointed Time: A Window of Opportunity

While often a static point in the future for most of us, our appointed time can be a moving target or a "window of opportunity," depending on whether we are "finished" with this life. It's the application of our free will that determines our final moments on Earth University.

I say *window* because the dying soul will sometimes wait for birthdays, holidays such as Christmas, daughters to graduate high school, or grandbabies to be born before we let go and pass over. This window can be hours, days, or months before death, but usually not more.

Since I have had so many premonitions of my death with the additional challenge of overcoming deadly brain cancer, I tell everyone that God will give me "just enough time to finish exactly what I need to do." I certainly want to be here for my kids; to see Angela graduate, to see Ben flourish, be with my wife and family, and I want to finish the *Chronicles* as I envisioned them to be written. My appointed time is set, and I may not have much choice in the matter.

Death with Dignity? Or is it suicide by another name?

Does God give us the free will to choose our time of death? Do we have the wisdom to choose? Is this an excuse for suicide? Perhaps, before we are born, God sets a pre-ordained "appointed" time of death. But this appointed time can become a bit blurry. Enter the case of Brittany Maynard, who had GBM IV, the same brain cancer I am walking through, who chose "Death with Dignity" —assisted suicide by taking a poison pill prescribed by her doctor. She set her own time of death on November 1, 2014—and stuck to her plan.

Brittany described her situation in an exclusive interview by *People Magazine*: *My glioblastoma is going to kill me, and that's out of my control," she told them. "I've discussed with many experts how I would die from it, and it's a terrible, terrible way to die. Being able to choose to go with dignity is less terrifying." After exploring and weighing the options available to her, Maynard and her husband decided to move from San Francisco to Portland, OR, where she would have access to Oregon's Death with Dignity Act (DWDA). Passed in 1997, the law "allows terminally-ill Oregonians to end their lives through the voluntary self-administration of lethal medications, expressly prescribed by a physician for that purpose.* [39]

Without getting into judgment regarding whether her choice was right or wrong, who can say that God did not plan for her to die on November 1, 2014, before she was born?

~I just heard Brittany Maynard took her life only two days ago on November 1st, just as she planned. She was 29. Upon reading the news, I broke out in tears. I didn't necessarily agree with her position, nor do I agree with the term "Death with Dignity," but I understand it.

---

[39] One Woman's Quest to Die with Dignity—and What It Means for Us All, *Ryan Wallace*, Oct 7, 2014

I know her decision to end her life on her terms, very, very deeply. In some ways, we GBM brain tumor "sufferers," while disconnected by distance and communication, still feel like a spiritual family, a sort of "volleyball team" that lost one of its team members. I was surprised how much I cried over her death. I prayed for her family, and I know for sure she is just fine in Heaven. She "chose" the time of her death and stuck to it. November 1, 2014...She had GBM much worse than I, with seizures nearly every day. ~**Chronicle 508**~

On March 24, 2015, my friend, Aaron Winborn, passed away. He'd decided to "pull the plug" after battling ALS for four years. I first met Aaron when he joined us at Hearthfire Lodge in Virginia in the late 1980s. While I studied under Paul Solomon, he became a student of the well-known expert in death and dying, Elisabeth Kübler-Ross, whose office and residence was only two hours south of Hearthfire.

The week prior, on March 18th, he had written a Facebook farewell letter to friends and family that included an invitation to his memorial service. *"Farewell, all my friends, old and new. I have decided to "pull the plug" on March 24. I have to say that these past 47 years have been a grand adventure, and it is bittersweet to see it end. It will be quick and painless, and I am at peace with my decision. I am sad that I'm leaving my family. Though these words don't adequately express my feelings, they're the best I have. To all of you who have been touched, no, mauled, by ALS, hang on; a cure is undoubtedly on its way. Alas, unless it comes in the next week, it's too late for me. I am nearly at the point where it is impossible to communicate, and if you know me, you know how much I love to talk when I have something on my mind.*

Speaking of which, there are a few things I'd like to say. First, I want to express my gratitude to everyone who has supported me and my family in a multitude of ways. You have made all the difference in the world, and I expect you'll have nothing but good karma coming your way. I wish I had the time and energy to thank each of you personally. Suffice to say, I thank you and I wish the best for you and yours. Next, I need to say that I will be spending the days I have left in solitude with Gwen, Ashlin, and Sabina. Although I will continue to read messages and emails, please don't expect a response.

I have such limited time and energy now, and I want to focus all of it on my family.

When I lived with Elisabeth Kübler-Ross some 27-years ago, I thought it odd that so many people would send her butterflies. I don't mean literal butterflies, but rather drawings and stuffed cushions shaped like butterflies, many of which were created by terminally ill patients. I used to think that they (butterflies) symbolized the notion of life after death. But now I've come to the conclusion that they actually represented the idea of life BEFORE death. This is an important distinction, one which I feel fortunate to have made before my end.

Thus the personal mantra that I've had these past few months, that goes something like, "6 more beautiful days, and today is the most beautiful yet.

Meryl Ann Butler, Managing Editor of *Oped News*[40] and long-time friend of Aaron's wrote: "Aaron was forty-seven and married with two little girls. Four years ago he was diagnosed with ALS (Amyotrophic Lateral Sclerosis, also known as Lou Gehrig's disease). He navigated a rapid deterioration with more grace and dignity than most people muster for dealing with daily stress. ALS is 100% fatal and results in a slow death, with the most common cause of death being suffocation resulting from a paralyzed diaphragm muscle. The disease afflicts about 350,000 people in the world annually. Approximately half of the patients die within three years of diagnosis."

Meryl Ann points out in her article, "After Aaron made his announcement, a few religious fundamentals rebuked him or tried to dissuade him, some even publicly suggested he had made a wrong choice and might be punished for eternity.

Thankfully, the vast majority of people posting on Aaron's and his family's Facebook pages were compassionate, understanding, and supportive and offered heartwarming words of comfort. He'd surrounded himself with an extended family of deep friendship. And they all stretched out their love to midwife him on his journey. Few on this planet have walked through the doorway to the beyond with the understanding, peace, and grace that Aaron exhibited in his life, and in his poignant final post on Facebook."

In closing, Aaron commented on Facebook about the process of dying he had experienced during the last four years. He said:

---

[40] *Meryl Ann Butler is an artist, author, educator and OpEdNews Managing Editor who has been actively engaged in utilizing the arts as stepping-stones toward joy-filled wellbeing for her entire professional career. She currently owns and operates Ocean View Arts in Norfolk, Virginia.*

First off, it's not a matter of dying, so much as a process of living. I can't stress that enough. Even if we haven't had the pleasure of meeting, I want to affirm how influential you have been in my life. I love life dearly, in all its forms. Thank you for indulging me these few, precious minutes.

Aaron asked to be taken off life support. It was his choice. It was between him and God.

Before his passing, Aaron wrote a book for his daughters. *Where did Daddy Go?* The book was published after his passing. He wanted to help his daughters understand and process his death. It is written from the perspective of a child.

Aaron, happy journeys. I'll miss you. It won't be so long until we get to "hug" each other in Heaven!

—— 16 ——

The Twister

The Zen of GBM

Dorothy Eadie, who wrote, *Embraced by the Light,* writes: *To my surprise, most of us had selected illnesses we would suffer, and for some, the illness that would end our lives. Sometimes healing does not come immediately, or at all, because of our need for growth. All experience is for good, and sometimes it takes what we would consider negative experience to help develop our spirits...*

The pain we experience on earth is just a moment, just a split second of consciousness in the spirit world, and we are very willing to endure it. Our deaths are also often calculated to help us grow. When a person dies of cancer, he may experience a long, painful death that may give him growth opportunities he cannot get otherwise.[41]

Both the caregiver and the dying grow spiritually from these challenges.

Diagnosis of a terminal illness is a difficult thing for my family and most people to accept. We don't want our loved ones to pass on unnaturally or, indeed, not too soon. Five months is too young. Five years is too young; 29 is too young, and 55 years is too young. Understandably, we want them to stay with us forever. We have a society of positive thinkers, believers who live by Faith, and a "you can do anything you set your mind to" people.

---

[41] Eadie, Dorothy J. 1992. *Embraced By The Light.* Placerville, CA: Gold Leaf Press. pp. 67-68.

As a terminally ill patient with GBM, I was subjected to sixty days of debilitating chemotherapy. My brain has been fried for thirty days, with intense radiation to kill cancer cells. Daily prescriptions keep swelling and seizures under control, lest I fall and crack my face on cement or have a stroke. I endure numerous blood tests, undergo every kind of medical examination you can imagine, and suffer through hours of MRI's like a caged animal--all in the effort to save my physical body from dying.

The terminally ill are repeatedly bombarded with well-intended proclaimations, "just have a positive attitude...you can fight this!" "Be strong for those that love you." "'There is a cure if you take this green herb, that homeopathy, or apply a magnetic helmet on your head."

Or simply, "Have faith God will heal you." At first, the cheerleading is fine, but after a year or two, it gets old. The question begs. Is it worth it? How much do I fight the process? Should I fight? Should I switch to a "prevent death at all costs" mode? The "fight" becomes more than physical. It becomes a mental, emotional, and spiritual battle fought on another field entirely and is as important as medical treatment.

I often read comments on brain cancer blog boards from caregivers of GBM loved ones or GBM sufferers who often describe the disease as --horrible, awful, horrendous --an ugly death. And as we read, even Brittany Menard took her own life six months early, afraid of the "terrible pain" she would experience during her last days.

And even though I saw my good friend quietly die of GBM in 2007, the same quiet ending for Delynn's mother Barbara in 1993, many GBM terminally ill patients die comfortably in the care of hospice, yet others do not. I think any illness that is bringing life to an end is awful, it's difficult, and we don't know how to handle it.

So, which is better? To die of a heart attack or accident that suddenly takes us away from our family with no warning with no time to say goodbye? I have sometimes thought about this myself. Gosh, wouldn't it be better just to drop dead from a heart attack? I sometimes despair of the constant daily struggle with GBM as there are no breaks. I desire to wake up feeling normal, and each day I wake up with that genuine hope.

In many ways, I am fortunate. I have not had much pain, but my life has been dramatically diminished. I can't drive long distances anymore. I can't bowl or golf anymore. Anything that requires balance or walking too far is a non-starter for me. I can speak, think, and write. I can still have a daily coherent conversation with my wife, children, mother, and sisters. There are still many things I can do. I can even shoot pool. I can float in the ocean, and when I float in water, gravity is removed from my tumor, and momentarily my wonky, equilibrium symptoms disappear. The doctors still can't figure that one out.

Interpretations of GBM as a horrific and terrible disease may be accurate from the caregiver's point of view, or terminally ill loved ones who are suffering or who are watching the suffering happen. Smelling and experiencing a septic tank doesn't make it any less awful to smell.

My experience with GBM is mixed. It has slowed me down and made me take a closer look at my life, relationships, and look at the mission I am supposed to complete, including healing my relationships with those in my life. On the other hand, it slows me down, dizziness, the ringing in my ears, the sensitivity to sound, and having this unrelenting need to complete my books.

If this disease or something like it didn't strike me down, I would have most likely avoided writing the Chronicles altogether. I know this for a fact because I had no plans to hurry the book along. On the other hand, GBM sometimes feels like slow torture.

It has completely dominated the life of my wife, Delynn, with its roller-coaster ups and downs. She stays on top of scheduling doctor appointments, blood tests, MRI's, ensuring they've actually been set and that my medicine will arrive on time. On top of that, she works as a secretary for the church, my business, and this book.

Every two months, we make our eight-hour round trip to Duke University, holding our breath to hear the MRI results. It seems endless, and sometimes I wish God would just get it over with. But I do believe it is essential I persist living as long as I can.

~Worked two hours on the "Zen of GBM" chapter. It was coming together nicely. Dr. Randazzo at Duke liked the chapter. Off in the golf cart to Nick's for breakfast. Forgot my wallet and couldn't pay the $6 bill. I told the waitress I would come back later to pay. I came back at noon to find out a Good Samaritan eating breakfast overheard I had forgotten my wallet and paid for my breakfast. No one had ever done that for me before. **~Chronicle 684**

~Today showed me the amazing hand of God. It was the first anniversary of my first GBM symptoms. An auspicious day. We moved into our new 3-bedroom apartment overlooking the ocean. A bit larger space and just in time for Angela to move into her new bedroom. Auspicious indeed. She arrives tonight on a late flight from Washington! And by the way, our apartment number is 433. It is the same number as the house I moved into on Coconut lane in 1970 when my family moved to Virginia Beach. 433 also adds up to 10. God, the great architect, was working overtime to communicate his love to my family.

~This 365th Chronicle, since the doctor said, "Mr. Solomon, we have found a mass in your brain." I can't believe a year has gone by and I am still here.

Since the white stallion dream a week ago, I noticed a distinct change in my attitude. My daughter's arrival was the shot of love and family I so desperately needed. Our apartment overlooking the ocean was a breath of salt air to calm my soul. The sun came up at 5:30 a.m., and sitting on the small deck facing the ocean, feeling the heat of the early morning sun on my face was heaven. I was beginning to feel "hope." Instead of resigning to my deadly fate, I wanted to live. ~

Chronicle 365

Since I was diagnosed with GBM, I was never really afraid of dying. I always knew this day would come, perhaps sooner than I wanted. However, the problem was that I had resigned myself to dying. Since leaving Akio, I hadn't been "acting" as if I wanted to live. My June 6th dream of the white stallion and the brilliant white light had changed my attitude and given me a new lease on life. Overnight I made a conscious decision to change my perspective. As a wise friend told me, "Eat a live frog. Eat two if you have to." So, I guess I began eating live frogs in a manner of speaking.

My close relationship with Jesus has never wavered, but sometimes I get lost in my illness, forget my walk with the Lord. I became numb. I let my condition control my joy. I needed an attitude adjustment. A year ago, Delynn had a dream about "Don't forget to press the Joy button." A simple saying, I should remember more often. Could it be that simple?

In the movie the Bucket List, Freeman repays Nicholson's generosity by teaching him that the love and life lessons we leave behind can be our most enduring and vital legacy.

As they overlook the Egyptian pyramids, Freeman tells Nicholson that, according to Egyptian lore, you're asked two questions at the gates of Heaven. How would our lives change if not just once but each time the sun sets? We asked these two questions:

Question 1: Did I experience joy today?

Question 2: Did I bring joy to someone else today? ~**Chronicle: 362**

GBM Survival Rates Improving

Since the U.S. Food and Drug Administration's approval of Temozolomide (Temozolomide) to treat adult patients with newly diagnosed glioblastoma (GBM) in 2005, the 24-month survival rate of glioblastoma patients has doubled, from 12% to about 25%. "Ten years ago, people were not talking about brain tumor survivorship issues," said John de Groot, M.D., an associate professor in the Department of Neuro-Oncology at The University of Texas MD Anderson Cancer Center. "But this new standard of care seems to have shifted the bar."

Despite this progress, nearly 100% of glioblastomas recur, usually within 6–8 months after ceasing treatment. The median survival duration of glioblastoma patients is 16–19 months; their 5-year survival rate is less than 10%.

"There's a sense of futility if you read the numbers. But statistics are just statistics; they mean nothing for the individual patient," Terri Armstrong, Ph.D., a professor and an advanced practice nurse in the Department of Neuro-Oncology, said. "Our approach to every glioblastoma patient is to control the tumor for as long as we can. It's something the person is going to be dealing with for the rest of his or her life, and our goal is to maximize the patient's treatment options and ability to function during that time."

There are many new "immune" therapies being employed in the US, UK, and Israel. There appear to be promising developments. All are in the Clinical Trial stage, with usually only a small handful qualifying for treatment.

When a tumor begins progressing, the fallback is still chemo and additional radiation if tolerated. While helpful to increase energy and stamina, diet and supplements have not shown to be of any consistent help to cure GBM due to its aggressive nature.

~We "GBM" survivors count our lives in months and days, not years. 33% suffer seizures. 33% have pain. Some have very little or no pain. At this point, I am one of the lucky ones. I have very little pain. Mostly 30-second "brain twitches" where my tumor is located. The pain can be intense for a few moments. The doctors don't know why I have them. The reality is I have a hand grenade, pin pulled, ready to go off in my brain. If the brain tumor doesn't kill me, seizures or strokes will. It's not a matter of if, but when. That's the reality. I know it. And so I do not waste time. I am either writing, doing a bit of business, or spending precious time with my family. ~**Chronicle 372**

Cheryl Boyle's 15 Year GBM Survivor story

In June 2000, Cheryl Broyles, 33 years old, was working in Oregon as a wildlife biologist with Threatened & Endangered Species, began having headaches that felt like her skull was going to explode. An MRI showed her brain was hemorrhaging, and she went into surgery at OHSU in Portland, Oregon. An acorn sized Glioblastoma Multiforme (GBM) tumor was found in her left temporal lobe. She was told she had less than a year to live. But as of 2015, she has become one of only a handful who has survived fifteen years.

In her blog, she writes about her 15-year GBM survivor story, especially about her brain fatigue vs. physical fatigue: *"Over the last 15 years of battling the Glioblastoma Multiforme, I realized that it is not just "physical" fatigue that hits us, patients. Yes, the chemo makes us weak and tired, but it is more than that. I've been off all treatment for three years ...and I still get VERY fatigued.*

I used to think of it mostly as "physical" fatigue because I would feel so worn out I would need to take a nap in the afternoon before my two boys got home from school. Some days I felt great and perky, with my brain working clear. Then another day I would feel fatigued and like a vegetable and would just curl up on the couch, not having energy to do anything. I was SO frustrated thinking "why do I have good days and bad days?"

Cheryl writes on her website, "*Then I started seeing a speech therapist (because I was having a harder time understanding what people were saying, because of background sounds distracting me). She gave me info that opened my eyes! The fatigue I was getting was not "physical" fatigue, but "brain" fatigue!!!! My neuro-oncologist told me years ago that my brain (after treatment damage) is like an 80+-year-old lady (I'm only 45). I remember wondering years ago why my grandma was always in her PJs by 4:00 p.m. in the afternoon, and she was too worn out to do much. Now I know why! Our brains get tired!!!! For us with brain tumors, and the damage from the tumor and the treatment, it makes it VERY difficult to do the normal "thinking."*

Reading her story helped me. Some days, I need complete silence for a few hours to recover from my brain's overstimulation.

In August 2015, Cheryl had her seventh recurrence of the GBM, a tiny inoperable 3.2mm tumor treated with Gamma Knife. On August 14th, Cheryl posted on Facebook a revelation about her recent GBM recurrence she titled "*The Finish Line*": "*In the past I have run many 5K races, Mt bike races, triathlons, x-country races, etc. And one of my favorite parts of the race is hitting the finish line!!! I love how I keep up my pace through the race and am even boosted to exceed and give it my ALL as I approach the finish line.*

What came to my mind as I drove past Mt Shasta was - I WILL continue to keep up my pace in life and never give up until I hit the finish line of life. I would not want to slow down and crawl to the finish line. I will not let this brain cancer and other worries of life drag me down to the ground, crawling to the finish line of my life. I will keep giving it my all!!!

The bottom line, Cheryl says, *"Don't give up hope. You are not a number in the statistics! Don't listen to the doctors if they tell you to go home and die. Plan to live and enjoy each second you have. Lean on God for strength and peace. He will always be there for you."* Cheryl's GBM story is updated periodically. http://www.cherylbroyles-gbm.com.

Seeking the Cure – Laying on Hands Healing

Some people have wondered why I haven't gone to more laying on hands healing services. In June 2014, my visit with Nigel Mumford in Virginia Beach ended with the laying on of hands recovering. I certainly can attest that his healing is likely one of the many reasons I am still here today. John of God is highly recommended in Brazil, but the cost of airfare and a "guide" to get us there was prohibitive. So I chose to stay home.

In some Christian sects, laying on hands healing is practiced quite regularly. It is not common, but a few ministers/preachers called to the healing ministry, lay hands on the forehead, often causing the person to be healed to "fall" unconscious to the floor. The Christian Term is "Slain in the Spirit."

When I traveled with Paul Solomon in the early 1980s, we did several healing tours throughout the northeast. Because of his reputation for healing, Paul would attract large crowds. Services would begin with an inspirational talk that prepared a person to "let go" of the disease.

Paul told them, "when I lay my hands on you, "let go and give him the disease." He said he would "absorb" the disease and then give it to God. And so he became a "conduit" of healing.

Services would begin with the entire audience singing *alleluia* for about five or ten minutes. A beautiful atmosphere of love and a Spirit of holiness filled the room. He then would begin calling for those wishing to be healed to come upfront. Paul embraced them, whispered in their ear a prayer, and then pressed his right hand on their forehead. Immediately, they would fall unconscious into the arms of a "catcher" standing ready behind them. Some would cry or laugh when they awoke. Sometimes more than a dozen would be lying on the floor, side by side, going through their healing experience.

I was one of the catchers. Young and strong, it was my job to lower the person carefully to the floor. I had to be quick because the line, sometimes more than a 100, would begin to pile up those "slain in the spirit" so fast, I could hardly keep up. Paul was scarcely conscious himself during the healing service, so I had to observe not to let someone fall to the floor without being caught.

I could feel the fire of the healing spirit coming from Paul, who would sweat so profusely his suit and shirt would be soaked after a service.

Healings did occur. One man gained his hearing. A few claimed they were cured of cancer. Many more were emotionally and mentally healed.

~Then it hit. The colon cramps, head-spinning, and before I knew it, an hour had gone by going back and forth to the bathroom. There would be no breakfast today. The colon pain has a domino effect on my entire body and brain. Nausea, and I for a few minutes, I forget I have brain cancer. How ironic. My brain tumor is killing me, but my colon is torturing me...to death. How stupid is that? **~Chronicle 818**

I'm sure it will be a while before my editors read these notes, and most likely it will be after I am gone (I hope I have to redact them later should I live longer than I expect), but I would rather be "real" than convey platonic nonsense.

A New Hope-Are we on the threshold of a cure for GBM?

After I stopped my chemo in September 2015, I wondered, "When will the inevitable progression of cancer begin?" Statistically, I am nearing the end of my rope. Less than 15% of GBM patients survive longer than three years. Will I be among the lucky 15%?

New cancer "cures" may be tipping the odds in my favor.

On March 29th, 2015, when I saw the CBS 60 Minutes special *"Use polio to treat cancer?"*—brain cancer, I was in tears from the very beginning of the show. I had been carrying the burden of survival for nearly two years, a yoke I required of myself to carry for God and family. After so many months of radiation and chemo, there now appeared new hope at Duke University with new clinical trials using Polio to destroy brain tumors. What? Seriously?

Yes. The doctors at Duke used a non-lethal form of the poliovirus engineered by molecular biologist and associate professor at Duke University, Matthias Gromeier. He had proved the genetically modified virus was safe after injecting the poliovirus into monkeys over seven years. In all that time, none of the monkeys contracted polio.

How did he achieve this feat? Gromeier removed the poliovirus's inherent disease-causing ability by splicing a piece of a cold genetic code, causing rhinovirus into the poliovirus genome. The result; the new PVS-RIPO kills cancer cells, but not normal cells with no ability to cause poliomyelitis and no ability of the PVS-RIPO to change back to a wild type of poliovirus that can cause poliomyelitis.

When Gromeier first introduced his idea to Doctor Henry Friedman, a leading neuro-oncologist and deputy director of the Brain Tumor Center at Duke University, he believed Gromeier was "nuts" -- that the notion polio might kill cancer tumors was insane. Friedman thought he was using a "weapon that produced paralysis." That was 15 years ago. After research, animal trials, and now this human clinical trial, they are more than optimistic. "This, to me, is the most promising therapy I have seen in my career, period." Friedman has been researching a cure for glioblastoma for more than 30 years.

How does it work? Gromeier explained how it works in the CBS 60 Minute interview, "All human cancers, they develop...protective measures that make them invisible to the immune system and this is precisely what we try to reverse with our virus," he says. "We are actually removing this protective shield...enabling the immune system to come in and attack."

Doctors believe the re-engineered poliovirus starts killing the tumor but that the body's own immune system does the real killing.

How effective is the new polio therapy? The first two patients who participated in the first clinical trial for the treatment in 2011 have been declared cancer-free by doctors.

60 Minutes cameras spent nearly a year chronicling the ups and downs of Duke's bold experiment. As the researchers struggled to determine how the virus would behave, their hard decisions sometimes led to tragic consequences for participating patients.

Early Phase I Polio clinical trials on Glioblastoma tumors experimented with different quantities of the Poliovirus, which is infused slowly through a needle drip over six hours directly into the tumor center. Doctors began increasing polio doses in the hope of a quicker result.

While early Phase I trials appear to have been a success, subsequent experiments with higher doses have been unsuccessful, with 11 patients succumbing to their disease.

But are the other eleven who were administered lower doses cured? That's what we are waiting to hear. Phase I trials are not usually successful. If the trials go well over the next twelve months, the program could receive "breakthrough" status, availing the therapy to more patients.

At the moment, I do not qualify to participate in the Phase I poliovirus trials at Duke University. Qualifications to enter the program require tumors to be larger than 1cm and smaller than 5cm. My 3mm tumor is currently too small and located too close to the midline of my brain. Why is that an issue? Because a poliovirus infusion would cause significant swelling of the tumor, possibly breaking the mid-line barrier – an often fatal development. The doctors at Duke do not have enough patient trials to understand how much the poliovirus is required. If the dosage is too high, it causes swelling and death.

Too little, and it doesn't work at all. Dr. Randazzo says (as of May 23, 2015) it's probably two years before the research yields enough clarity in dosage and results before they risk it with me.

Can I survive another twenty-four months to receive this proven polio viral treatment when it is more widely available? Statistically, for me, it's a long shot. But I am not a statistic.

Miraculous Healings at death's door

So, while I survive another year and wait for the poliovirus "cure," what other avenues of healing are available to me? Earlier in the chapter, I related the miraculous death door healing of Reverend Nigel Mumford, the story Hospice chaplain Dick Dingus shares the same experience. And here are a few more:

Cheri had a heart attack, and the doctors were unable to restart it for several minutes. As she drifted off to another dimension, her life review helped her understand her sickness and how to heal herself: *I was able to understand why I had become sick through my life review. And I was able to see exactly what energy or belief was being held within my spiritual vibration that was being carried from lifetime to lifetime or dimension to dimension. It was very clear. I knew what it was I needed to do in this lifetime to clear that energy so my spirit no longer has to carry that suffering into another lifetime."* [42]

Malla begs God for healing: *God, how can you leave me like this?' I sobbed. 'Have I not tried to live by your principles?' 'Have I not been good?' 'Huh? Have I not, God?' I rambled on. 'Ok, I'm not perfect, but no one is! I'm just human for f@#$'s sake! If you are all that grand and loving, why don't you end this terrible suffering I'm in?' The feeling of disillusion was growing inside of me as I grew more and more agitated. My mind was still convincing me that I was a victim of my own experiences. I was not able to understand that the outcome of my life was solely in my own hands. The pain and despair I was constantly engulfed in, was overwhelming. Not only was I breaking down physically, I was very much on the edge of complete mental breakdown. My body was literally beating me up to the point that I was dying. I had no life left and death did not want me.*

I did not know how to choose a new way of living my life. God, or someone at least, was trying to show me a way [she thought]. If this is real, I need to wake up and realize that this is my life. I decide. It is my choice; I am not a puppet in strings. I am in charge of my own destiny. 'If this is real,' I thought, 'We've got God all wrong. Not only do we have God all wrong, but we've also got ourselves all wrong!'

---

[42] *Cheri B's NDE*, #2969, 03.01.12, NDERF.org

If I want to die, convinced that there is no other way of continuing my physical existence; I will create my way out of here and there is absolutely nothing wrong with that. I will do this easily, by engaging in negative beliefs and experiences about myself and my life, leading to an illness or an accident that eventually will bring me to my death. If I fear that suffering is necessary in the process of living and that life is hard; it will be. All I have to do is to realize that I do not have to die in order to live. Whether we choose to live to live or die to live, the outcome is the same. Life!"[43]

The magic of "seeing" the truth of our lives while suspended in another dimension beyond the veil is at once exciting and yet still a mystery. Saint Anita, Saint Nigel, Saint Cheri, and Saint Malla all describe the clear realization about their "beliefs" and their "state of mind," which hold the secret to true healing - from a Heavenly perspective.

It is still the ultimate challenge for those looking for a miracle to heal our sickness on Earth. The old adage, "Healer, heal thyself," applies here. It sounds nice, but while we are caught up in the pain and illness, the reality of health seems remote. The ideal of healing seems philosophically sound, but the real-life application is a different story when you are sick. Jesus hinted, "It was their faith that made them whole" when miraculous healings occurred.

Faith. It's not a matter of trying. As Yoda said, "Try not. Do!"

Scott shares his thoughts: *Then, I heard a voice that called me. It was a male voice, firm and loving. He said that my mission had been accomplished. I let myself go; I wished to be there for the eternity, I didn't want to come back.*

---

[43] *Malla's possible* NDE/STE from a nurse, #3933, 04.27.15, NDERF.org

He said: I am going to show you some things. Then, in the distance, I saw a globe that looked like the moon during an eclipse. He said: That is the Earth, and I saw many points of light in the globe. Then He said: in every point of light there is someone praying, if all the people on Earth could pray, it would look like that, and the Earth became illuminated as the sun. But so is not and the globe darkened again. [44]

The challenge of overcoming an imminent prognosis of death reverts to faith in God—and a request for the miraculous to happen. Faith and the power of prayer have been a stumbling block for me since I was young. I admit that. Even though I was supposed to believe in prayer, I wanted to believe and would pray, God, I wasn't always sure the effect prayer would have on those who needed help. It was a spiritual act that required faith that something real was happening. When I was diagnosed with brain cancer, many friends and family worldwide began praying for me. They put me in a circle and prayed for me, which I appreciated, but it was very awkward. I wanted to run and hide. I did not want to be the center of attention. In truth, I didn't know how to accept love.

~I goofed off today and watched the movie "in Time." The message I got from the film, 'Do not waste my time!' It's God's time, not my time.

~Chronicle 784

Prayer and faith are connected like twin souls.

Dennis, an internet gold blogging acquaintance, who became my friend, emailed me about his wife's experience being cured of brain cancer by faith. I was thankful for her healing. One day she went in for an MRI, and the tumor was suddenly gone. It was a miracle. Gone. The doctors couldn't explain it or even want to talk about it.

---

[44] *Scott H NDE, #2698, 05.02.11, NDERF.org*

Dennis explained to me that God ordained that we live to seventy. Well, explain that to a mother whose child died in their teens. Was it the sin of the mother or the child's to die before seventy years of age? I think we all have an ordained time, but many grey lines are crossed when we become ill.

Fanny saw the power of prayer from her Heavenly perspective: *It was certain time after, while I was in the ICU, I remember my body lying, left "to die" like if it was my funeral. It was dark all around I actually thought, "now they are waiting for me to die" But at the same time I was looking at myself, and I looked like my father when he died. I remember realizing this similarity, and being aware of the situation, thinking about it. "this is my funeral," I thought, I was floating in the air and, far to the right, I could see thousands of beings coming towards me, each one carrying a little light. These beings were coming from different parts of the world to like pray for me, for my life. And I could feel the energy, the love? And I was attending to what was happening."*[45]

~I was reading that some GBM terminally ill patients begin sleeping a lot – like 16-20 hours a day – during the last 4 to 8 weeks of life. I have often felt fatigued and extremely dizzy in the afternoons over the previous four weeks and have needed to rest on my back and close my eyes.

I feel pressure on my left eyeball, the left side of my head at the base of my skull, and the upper left neck area, where the tumor is located.

It is difficult to sit up for any length of time or walk any distance more than 100 yards without feeling disoriented. So I lie down. The intensity of my disorientation makes me wonder if the tumor is progressing. I've been wrong before.

---

[45] Fanny P's Probable NDE, #2422, 10.11.10, NDERF.org

It could be the prednisone or Ambien side effects. It is commonly reported that as GBM patients lower their steroid doses, they often lose their ability to walk and talk. It's such a friggen crapshoot. I just want to feel better. ~**Chronicle 819**

When I started this GBM journey, extending my life two years seemed far-fetched. I honestly didn't think it would happen. On September 29, 2014, I had a dream about expecting unfaithful waters. I need to trust that God will give me exactly the amount of time, energy, and health. I need to finish my mission on Earth.

Perhaps living or dying is about arriving at our "appointed time" and fulfilling our life mission. Could it be as simple as life wrapped up like a box of chocolates, never knowing what we will get? When Forrest Gump's mother told Forrest she was dying, she said, "Forrest, it's my time." She smiled at him, "Forrest, death is a part of life." Doctors who are desperately trying to prolong or keep "alive" a terminally ill patient should attempt to listen to the dying patient and their heart and appreciate the insight. It is not a failure. It is their "time." We can do all we believe with help our loved one stay with us, including the best vitamin therapies; the best medical care; access to clinical trials, and raised money to receive highly potent, curative vaccines, but when it is someone's "time" to leave Earth University, nothing can stand in the way of their death.

It may be a simple truth. However, most of the time, we don't accept it because we are often unwilling to face death. We turn away from it and, in the process, often lay judgments and expectations on the terminally ill patient.

As I continue my journey through this illness, I pray my experiences have found a place in your heart and mind.

As much as we sometimes yearn for our lives to stay the same, they do not. At the very best, we are blessed to grow older each day with the people we love. We are equally blessed if we can grow wiser from our past experiences, not just the good ones but also the bad ones.

I have learned that as our lives evolve and unfold in ways we could have never imagined, in the end, we must always find peace both within ourselves and with our lives. I will forever have a two-inch scar on the back of my head. My tolerance for my daily wonkiness, my unstable gate, and dizziness continues unabated. I will be monitored with MRI scans every two months for the rest of my life since there is a high probability that my tumor will begin growing again.

Like Brittany, most people will never know just by looking at me; I even have a brain tumor. But whether I look like I have a brain tumor or not (what does a person with a brain tumor look like anyway?), one thing is for sure is I am truly blessed. I am forever changed because of my new perspective, deepened empathy, renewed faith, and extreme gratitude for life.

What is the Zen of GBM? The taste of ice cream when you are sick. With Caramel.

~Dead Saint Experiences and dreams are not the whole truth. Even the Apostle Paul admitted his experiences were only "known in part." Encounters with the afterlife are interpreted by the Saint's belief structure and expertise. Yet, the cumulative effect of anecdotal evidence should not be dismissed lightly. ~**Chronicle 367 (06.15.14)**

17

The Trenches

Reporting "Live" from the Afterlife Foxhole

"To everything, there is a purpose under Heaven, a time to live, and a time to die." Ecclesiastes 3:1-2

British physicist Sir William Barrett published "Deathbed Visions," a full-scale study of visions patients received before their final moments of death. He discovered dying is more frightening to the onlookers than it is to the patients themselves. While most dying patients drift into "oblivion" without awareness of it, there are some who are conscious to the end, who say they can "see" into the beyond, and who can report their experiences before expiring. Osis and Haraldsson's research, published *"At The Hour of Death,"*…among 10% of patients who were conscious in the hour before death, a few experienced vivid visions, often entailing graphic descriptions of the world to come, visitations with deceased relatives, encounters with great light, and a profound sense of serenity.

~I have observed GBM is slowly eroding at my ability to be 'present.' I am spilling water and banging and bruising my knuckles more often. I am losing awareness of exactly where my hands are. I have lost feeling inside my lower right shin down to my foot. I can still walk because my right thigh is not numb. My thigh just lifts the "wooden leg." I can still walk, but I have to be conscious of lifting my right foot over bumps and carpet edges. Everyone worries about me falling. My T'ai Chi training has come in handy, managing balance, and keeping my weight centered and low; otherwise, I would have certainly tripped and fallen by now. ~ **Chronicle 985** February 22, 2016

~It has been getting more challenging to walk every day. It was especially noticeable when Delynn tried to walk me upstairs to take a shower. With each step upstairs, my right foot banged against the stairs like a wooden log. Notwithstanding my disorientation and dizziness, I can barely lift my right leg and tell the difference from walking upstairs just three days ago.

Delynn had improvised a shower chair (actually my chair/urinal potty) to be placed firmly in the tub so that I could sit down, and she could safely wash my hair and wash me with soap without me falling. Just five weeks ago, my living quarters were the master bedroom upstairs. I took a shower every day on my own. But since my seizure on January 16th, 2016, Delynn made the living room downstairs our master bedroom. We do not have a shower downstairs.

I was trying to sit on the shower chair carefully when my right foot began twitching once per second. I looked at Delynn and grinned, "Seizure break." I breathed to relax. No big deal. Dr. Gupta told me my seizures would probably not be grand mal seizures, where I would collapse, go into contortions, bite my tongue, pee all over myself, and lose consciousness and possibly die from an aneurysm.

Not today.

Today is February 25, so it is precisely 40 days since my last seizure. Well, at least God has a sense of humor. 40 days-between twitches. LOL.

This will most likely be my last shower upstairs.

Step by step, GBM has progressed enough to change my daily life, but we had a contingency.

So as of today, I HAVE OFFICIALLY BECOME AHAB, THE MAN WITH THE WOODEN LEG! NOT FROM A WHALE BITE, BUT FROM A 25MM LEFT HEMISPHERE TUMOR SHUTTING DOWN THE NERVE SIGNALS TO MY LEG! ~Chronicle 988

~Talked to Delynn last night about triage. She said, 'What do you mean by that?' I responded, "When there is a disaster involving dozens of life-threatening injuries, doctors need to make quick decisions about who they will treat first. Those considered too far gone are treated last. The patients they think they can save are treated first. I realized today I needed to go into Triage mode to finish the Armageddon Stones. I will not have time to include all of my original ideas. Several chapters need to be condensed or re-written, and a few chapters eliminated. Such Triage will force me to write a better, focused book." February 28, 2016, **~Chronicle 991**

~After Mel, the Hospice nurse, left yesterday, it was official. I was dying. The reality of the moment was sobering. How did it make me feel? At this point, almost everyone wants to know: How much time do you have left? I can see the nearly daily decline in my strength. Who knows? I've had my dreams, but wake up at 4:00 a.m. and work on the Armageddon Stones until 11:00 p.m. at night. Another two to three weeks and the bulk of the writing will be done. Whatever is left to finish can be complete by a co-author over the summer.

How do I feel?

I feel like the Blue-eyed Duke Leto Atreides, Muad 'Dib, (Arabic – the teacher of literature), the Prophet in Frank Herbert's, Dune, who has gone as far as he can on his own will. Leto could not see the future anymore. It was a wall he could not see beyond. To move beyond it, to even live, he had no choice but to drink the Worm Drug Melange, the poisonous "water of life," the most important and valuable substance in the universe.

The poisonous Melange spice I needed to drink is understanding the mystery of God's preferred path for me. Will it come down to the last moment of my life, and Nigel Mumford is giving me the last rites before God and I come to a new agreement?

Do I accept the poison of death when all my body functions cease as my brain tumor shuts down my body? March 3, 2016~**Chronicle 995**

Delynn's notes: March 3rd is the same day David has his interview with Grimarica. He does not mention he'd just started hospice. That day I remember trying to keep him from writing or doing any work that would deplete his energy. The interview with Grim was in the evening, and David would typically be asleep by 7:00 p.m. He did rest, but as soon as I left to run to the market and was gone less than an hour when I returned, he had used his flipchart to write down all his notes.

I remember March 11th was the last day David walked outside with some help, and we went to Nick's restaurant. I remember this day because my son, James, was visiting and he had to leave that day.

~Paul Solomon died 22 years today, March 5, 1994. I have been up since 3:30 a.m. composing this strange introduction, knowing it will be published after my death. It is stranger still because, if the Lord gives me the honor of dying on the Lord's DAY of resurrection on March 27, if indeed, if that date is my dying date, then I have 22 days left to live. The number 22 is symbolic of the 22 paths of the Tree of Life. How woo woo is that? I can barely walk now or sit up now. I am bedridden. Delynn ordered Hospice (Bed) two days ago, so everything is set for my graduation from this life. Vol. II of the Chronicles, Training Wires of Soul, is complete. Vol III. of the Chronicles, The Armageddon Stones, are two weeks away from completion. But March 27th is Chronicle 1019, far short of my goal of 1101 days to see Angela graduate from High School on June 18, 2016, March 5, 2016 ~**Chronicle 997**

~4:30 p.m. Dick Dingus, Hospice Chaplin, comes for a formal visit. He played his guitar while handing me files to go through. After an hour of pulling out my 20-year-old Armageddon Stone research, we started talking about near-death experiences. Dick is a long time VB IANDS member and is quite knowledgeable about NDEs. Anyway, he describes the Dead Saint, who, on their deathbed, rises out of their body. He meets an angel who tells him it's his time to die, that his son will be okay and will be cared for. It stops him. Somebody else is going to take care of my son. I am going back. The angel insisted, 'no, it's your time now.' Back and forth they went until the Saint exasperated said, "You get Jesus down here right now, and we'll decide this. The angel said, "I will go talk to the boss." It wasn't long before the angel came back and said, your request to return is granted. But we want you to know your son will not learn the lessons he needs to learn with you there.

He looks down, and from his new perspective, heals the disease killing him. He, now, travels all over the world, telling them about the NDE that healed him.

Great story. I told him I had a few examples of these miraculous healings in the books. So with that, Dick said, "Let's pray." We prayed for healing for my leg so that I might walk again. During the prayer, he invoked God's golden light.

Suddenly, for a split moment, I found myself in the Sanctuary of Sekhmet in Karnak, Egypt, looking at Sekhmet face to face just as the picture shows. I had been there before in 2009 with John Anthony West. It was real. I was there for a moment. And just as suddenly, I was back holding hands, finish the prayer with Dick and Delynn. Dick just smiled and said, "Anything else?" without expecting an answer, he left.

We'd had several visitors with whom we'd have the discussion on dying, choices, and healing, whether considered from ourselves or a decision from God, when Delynn said, "David, why don't you just heal yourself? I told her, "It's not that simple. I need to have an NDE and get out of the body, where I can look into my brain, and from that perspective, along with God, do exactly the same thing. Could it happen to me? I looked at Delynn, "I've already had several discussions with God about this. Why write these books and then die, never really having a chance to preach the Chronicles to the masses, where I can make a difference?"

Dannion Brinkley had previously told me he believes something like a last-minute resurrection could heal me. On July 16, 2013, Angela's dream suggested I may be alive and healthy after three years.

God, I am sure you are listening. Guess I also have the attention of God's daughter Sekhmet.

To all my Christian friends, hey, I never even considered such an Egyptian help. Usually, it's just Jesus and me. Sure looks like He is okay with Sekmet as a Healing Ally. ~March 6, 2016, Chronicle 999

Sat, March 12th Peeing every 15 minutes. Waking up all night every 10 minutes. Paul Michels is coming over at 2 p.m. Chronicle 1003

On March 14, 2016, I awoke to realize the meaning of a dream of the past I had on July 15, 2013, just over a month after my GBM diagnosis. The dream described incidents leading up to the moment to terminate my own life:

I was in the ocean surf in Kauai, Hawaii. I was hit by a large wave and pushed hard towards the shoreline. I knew the shoreline represented Heaven. I heard someone yell from behind me that "three more waves are coming."

The first massive wave was the discovery of my Brain Cancer. The following three waves were symbolic. They represented my three books: Zen Journey through the Christian Afterlife, Training Wires of the Soul, and the Armageddon Stones. After the last book, represented by the third wave, was completed, it would push me ashore to Heaven.

Hospital Bed ordered and delivered today. I cannot lift myself. I can't stand or hold up my weight. Delynn called Heartland Hospice and ordered a motorized Hospital Bed. When it arrived, Delynn asked, "David, are you excited about dying?" No. I am tired of dying. I need a break. (Delynn: I know it probably sounds like a weird question for me to ask, but since we had been facing, writing, teach, speaking of this coming transition for nearly three years and having listened to death and dying antidotes daily and about the beauty of the life after this, it seemed reasonable for me to ask it.)

Another week's work on the Armageddon Stones, and then I am done. A co-author can finish the rest later ~**Chronicle 1005**

Bruce and Marty came to visit after hearing of David's decline. Bruce heads up most of the work at the church; he is a psychiatrist, counsel, and Marty, an oncology RN. They had been there to counsel us during some difficult family times and now the coming transition and challenges we were facing. We shared all of our current issues and needs. He quickly mobilized the members to assist in bringing daily one meal a day and, if available, an hour or two to allow Delynn to run errands.

March 15th, 2015

Hello Everyone,

David and Delynn have informed me that they would be most appreciative if we could schedule volunteers to visit with David each day to provide a luncheon meal for both David and Delynn.

Delynn is David's primary caregiver and has recently been feeling considerable fatigue and stress in her 24 hours per day's efforts to serve David. During the past week, David's physical health has deteriorated substantially; he informed me today when I visited with him that he is now unable to get out of his bed unassisted. He feels that he will be leaving us in the near future.

Now is the time for us to step forward to offer both David and Delynn our loving assistance. Our objective is to provide both David and Delynn a luncheon meal each day during the next three weeks (the schedule will then be extended as necessary).

If you feel inspired to be a part of this service project, please let me know what date(s) you would like to volunteer. Specifically, we are looking for volunteers on all dates beginning March 16th and ending April 5th. Please also provide me with alternate date(s) in case someone else picks the same date that you have selected. I will maintain a master schedule which I will send to all volunteers after it is established.

Delynn says that meals can be brought to their home anytime between 12-1:30 p.m. there are no dietary restrictions in terms of the types of meals that you would like to bring. Delynn says that David enjoys both vegetarian and meat dishes.

Delynn advises that they also have food available in their kitchen that a volunteer can prepare if they so desire. If you are interested in this option, simply call Delynn and she can let you know what food is available in their kitchen for you to prepare.

We are also looking for volunteers who are willing to spend 2-4 hours at the Solomon residence for the purpose of allowing Delynn to run errands and to have a rest period. If you're interested in assisting in this way, please call Delynn directly to arrange a date for your service.

This is what a spiritual Community is all about-assisting each other in times of need. I look forward to hearing back from you on this very important project.

Much love to everyone,

Bruce

~Dream: I heard: "The Word of God is Honey." Scripture truly is honey. Everyone wants to know how long I think I will live. I really don't know, but my brain is getting tired. Not long. Maybe three weeks or less. I feel weaker every day. Maybe March 27; ~**Chronicle 1006**

March 15, 2016, 9:28 p.m. Thank you everyone for your support, especially your thoughts and prayers. Any help will help, no matter how small. Sometimes just showing up for 30 minutes to help straighten up the kitchen, or maybe nothing at all, or to let me run to the bank, etc...some days seem more overwhelming than others. And today David's mom brought enough food for a few days. So...we are good for a few days on food. Also, my family will be here Easter weekend and we will not need help over that weekend.

Heartland Hospice already has been awesome. It has been an incredible blessing to have Dick Dinges come with hospice. He sometimes just comes and sits and sings and plays his guitar while David closes his eyes.

David would love to have visits. Typically only a 30 minute visit and then he gets tired. You are welcome to come even if my family is here.

We have sent David's book to print today. It takes a load off but now we shoot for all the media stuff. There is so much going on. David has been amazing. His mind is way beyond his body. I believe your thoughts, prayers, visits, etc...will carry him further!!

Also, on a practical side, I am overwhelmed with so many decisions/things we are working on/learning curves (business, books, medical, etc...) that to make a decisions on food/time/help/etc...can throw me over the top. I don't always know what I need or the time I will need it. Honestly, I cry everyday - at some point in the day. And I laugh. So do what it is in your heart to do, even if just to pray and be led by that. Yes, a little notice helps and...the side door is always open. Come on in...any time after 8:00 a.m. Just announce yourself when you come into the kitchen. LOL!

With love and sincere gratitude, - We miss you all!

Delynn

The emails flooded in, and in no time, three weeks of food and visits were scheduled.

~Dream: the word THE was missing from the Chronicle Printer Proof.

We had to decide to get a hard printer's proof. Dottie recommended it. And I still wanted to make edits. Instead, Delynn went to Kinkos and had the proof printed out. Getting an overnight hard proof would add five days to print. Delynn was afraid I would die before then. She is at the beach, reading our hard print to help us make a decision.

Delynn notes: I remember saying to David, in front of his mother, who was over that day, "David, if we have any more delays, you may die before we get your book printed; I know we have more edits and changes that could be made, but if you want to see your book I feel we should send it now."

Today is March 16, 2016. We had a big celebration yesterday; the final proof of that *Dead Saints Chronicles: A Zen Journey Through The Christian Afterlife* was sent to the printer. We did a big champagne opening with Skip, Delynn, Dawana, myself, and Ben and celebrated this momentous moment. It certainly took longer than we thought. I'm hardly able to set up, but I can drink a glass of champagne; it's one of those stress relievers. Now it's gone to the printer and is expected to be done on either April 4 or 5. We are in such a rush we will not be able to make available advanced orders by March 25, but we have to work with Dottie to have a rollout plan of what we're going to do if we are going to do a book signing. We have to offer something to have an initial purchase of books. Odyssey magazine has agreed to look at my articles; they may have a special toward the end of March, which works out perfectly. Graham Hancock will be featuring the Chronicles as the book of the month, April 1. I have an appointment to speak at the Casey Foundation, the A.R.E., on April 9. The challenge will be that I can't lift myself, and I can't go anywhere, so they're trying to work out a Skype or live stream so that I can give the talk. I hope they can do it. I hope

I'm still here to do it. Delynn did a YouTube of her new hospice wheelchair-bound shower technique and, within minutes, was put on YouTube. Delynn put up her own YouTube site last night. It's well done, so I hope it gets the following we want and let Dannion Brinkley know as well because he has 5500 VA hospice worker who would love to use the sample as an inexpensive technique.

Its greater purpose is for hospice workers. It's is a stroke of genius. Delynn's idea may make a difference for the Chronicles than anything else I can think of; who knows?

~So much is going on every day; it's almost hard to keep up my journal notes. I wanted to use today to finish book II. Thank you, Paul Michels, for this beautiful Apple notepad!! March 16, 2016. ~**Chronicle 1007**

Flashback: Stepfather Ray's Death June 18, 2015

Before I begin to talk about my own death, I want to flashback nine months ago to June 18, 2015, when my step-father, Ray, died during the writing of the final chapter of Vol. II, "A Time to Die," a chapter that was supposed to be about my own death. It became clear to me that somehow, we were bonded together in our transition and for the sake of my mother, who lost her husband of 29 years, and now was losing her son, only 57. So, Mom, I know that God will not give you more than you can endure, and still, I know the pain will seem too much at times to bear, along with the sadness. I can only try to shine the light of hope that we will all see each other soon in paradise.

I have been admitted to Hospice, showing every sign I am 4-6 weeks away from passing over. So follow along with Ray and me. I will start with Ray.

Ray began his transition to the other side around June 3, 2015. Ray was supposed to recover in the hospital, but the doctors sent him home to be treated in palliative care. On Sunday, June 7, the doctors sent Ray home in a Medical Transport. A hospital bed had been set up in the lower, downstairs den so Ray could be transported to his bed through the garage, and if needed, brought back and forth to the hospital to receive his kidney dialysis. Mom was not taking any more chances of a fatal fall down the stairs.

Ray had worked for NASA for nearly forty years. He was a brilliant man who did not have a degree in science. However, he still had been a valued member of NASA for his ability to solve challenging, electrical/mechanical problems that degreed associates couldn't figure out. Ray loved Star Trek and was indeed a man of science.

I knew Ray for 29 years since he married my mother. Most of that time, I was either gone traveling, building a company, or raising a family in Washington State on the other side of the country. We did not see each other much. I never really got to know him that well. He was a serious but happy person. He was a devoted family man who was deeply wounded by the tragic, untimely deaths of his daughter Susan and his grandson Daniel a decade earlier. He was a man of faith and prayer and wanted to be remembered as a "good man." Isn't that all the Lord requires of us? In Micah 6:8, the Word says, "To act and to love mercy and to walk humbly with your God." Ray Gregory exemplified these spiritual qualities his entire life.

When my wife, Delynn, and I moved from Washington State back to Virginia Beach a year and a half ago, I got to know Ray a lot better because we both had a common problem. We were both sick. His heart and kidneys were failing, and I had terminal brain cancer. When we looked at each other in the eye and didn't see it before, I saw his deep compassion, and I believe he saw mine. It was love. Just love. An understanding between us that went deeper than simple platitudes.

I had spent a bit more time with Ray over the past two months after a fall or two that sent him to the hospital. I gave him a little red rock engraved with the word "TRUST." A stone that meant in my mind "trust in the Lord." Mom said it meant a lot to him. And I am so thankful it did.

I could still see Ray was not ready to leave this life. I think it is why he fought so long to stay alive. But now he seemed to slip in and out of consciousness, showing symptoms almost like dementia. His care became more demanding.

At times I felt I was dying right along with Ray though there were no signs of the cancer growing. I would get exhausted and depressed from the effects of the tumor and drugs. I would talk about my end days. I sounded like I was ready to go and that we needed to prepare. Delynn became frustrated and yelled and cried, asking me not to talk about it when I was not close to dying. I was still doing well simultaneously, Ray was in hospice care and days from dying. It overwhelmed her to think about it because she knew what it would take to care of me when the time came. She reasoned why we would put the focus on it when it isn't happening. There would be a time when it was time, and the time was not now. It was difficult.

Delynn would take her regular breaks. Once I was asleep or would be writing and needed quiet, which was most of the time. She would go to her dream class, church, but mainly with her girlfriends, hoping to release the day's stresses. I was always writing and talking about death and dying while I was dying. Besides helping me with the businesses, writing, or working at the church, she helped with my teenage daughter's school enrollment, classes, dental and health issues. I was unable to do any of these things, including helping my daughter with her own struggles, including the idea of losing her father.

Delynn and I had church responsibilities since I'd decided to be on the board, and she helped in the office. We were trying to create a new ISO in the credit card business since my non-compete was up. She helped me keep track of my consulting work (listening in, managing, in case I missed things because I was in brain fog), all this plus managing the plethora of medical issues for me.

Who has been trained to deal with it, especially while all I write about is death and dying – it has been the central focus of my life for three years, and here I am closer than I ever thought I'd be. It's an ordeal. Handling a dying patient is a struggle. It is more than hard work; it's all-consuming and creeps into every corner of your life.

Mom, Ray's daughter, and my sister bore much of the burden of care for the last few weeks, bonding the whole family closer. Sometimes death does that, and it is beautiful to see. Family help when death comes is so essential.

Ray passed away Wednesday, June 18, 2015

Sometimes death wounds us for a long time. Grief is part of the process of losing a loved one. The pain will diminish with time, but it never really leaves. Elizabeth Kübler-Ross and John Kessler, both experts on death and dying, say, "The reality is that you will grieve forever. You will not 'get over' the loss of a loved one; you will learn to live with it. You will heal, and you will rebuild yourself around the loss you have suffered. You will be whole again, but you will never be the same. Nor should you be the same, nor would you want to."

When death breaks the emotional and physical bonds of life, it cuts us. Ecclesiastes 12:6-7 says, Remember him - before the silver cord is severed, or the golden bowl is broken; before the pitcher is shattered at the spring or the wheel is broken at the well, and the dust returns to the ground it came from, and the spirit returns to God who gave it."

Death is compared to cutting this cord and the crashing of the bowl down to the ground, whereupon it shatters, and its light extinguished. Ray's light was put out in this world and born again shining in the next.

We want to know, "Is Heaven for real?" Do our loved ones live on?

ADC Dream of Ray June 19

On June 19, a day after Ray died, I prayed intensely for my stepfather. I said, "Ray, this is your service, so if you want me to give a message of importance, you got to let me know." So, in the middle of the night, about 3:00 a.m., Ray suddenly appeared to me in a dream. It was not a usual kind of dream; it was like he was there. It was real. Everything was brightly lit behind him. And he was beaming! Every part of his face was smiling. His eyes sparkled. He looked 30 years younger. I don't think I have ever seen anyone so happy.

He did have a simple message he wanted me to tell you. It was apparent he was alive and that he was ok. The message was that we must love one another even more because nothing matters more than love.

You see, I believe, after death, when we approach the gates of Heaven, God will ask each of us a simple question, "Have you loved one another?"

I believe Ray will be able to humbly say, Lord, I have helped the unfortunate. I have been fair, faithful, and good. I have not been a perfect man, but I have been a loving man.

God judges us by the love in our hearts. Jesus says in Mark 12:30, "Love the Lord your God with all your heart and with all your soul and with all your mind and with all your strength." The second is this: 'Love your neighbor as yourself.' There is no commandment greater than these."

I told mom about my dream. She instantly knew it was real, broke down, and cried. Ray was alright. He was happy. He was alive.

He is in Heaven.

Then how should we think of Ray? He is not dead. He is alive, born again into his new immortal, spiritual body and released from the pains of this life.

I found it ironic that my first Sermon 31 years ago was at the funeral of my mother's second husband, Jack Sutton, who was killed in a tragic accident in 1984. Thirty-one years later, I presided over another funeral for her husband, Ray. She was worried I might not be strong enough to do it. I felt I owed to him, especially since he had the audacity to visit me in my dream and let me know he was happy and alive!

We visited the funeral home together. There are always so many decisions to make, a lot of paperwork, death certificates, decisions on casket type to cremation, clothing apparel, and so on. The girl in charge of the entire process, we nicknamed Morticia, a character's from the Adam's Family. She was weird but did a great job managing the funeral. It made me think of my own choices for cremation at my funeral – kind of a preview of what I might soon be experiencing myself. It felt creepy.

The next day I gave the best sermon I could muster. I had always wondered if I would die first and then be the soul escort for Ray at his death. But now it appears, Ray will be at my passing to escort me to Heaven. I shared my dream of Ray visiting me from the Afterlife. I know he came to me because he wanted to give Mom and the family reassurance life goes after the body.

Beyond that, I TRUST God believed his visit would make a monumental difference for you and me. Ray did not know I was writing this chapter in the book when he died, but his death punctuated his life and made a massive difference in my life, this book, and the lives of our friends and family.

It was a beautiful day, Remembrance of Ray, especially when my nephew, Joshua, gave his eulogy that was touching, funny, and real.

You never know why God does what He does. Or why God takes a loved one away and when. We just have to trust Him—for everything happens in its time, even death.

Mom, It's My Time

Back to the present, March 13, 2016. I felt it important to tie my passing with my stepfather Ray. I am borrowing all of his final dying week's equipment: potty chair, walker, and wheelchair. Like Ray, hospice is setup. We chose Heartland Hospice. Mel and Celeste visit me twice a week to shower me and check on my vitals. Dick Dingus is the Heartland Hospice Pastor and a long-standing pastor at the Fellowship of the Inner Light in Virginia Beach, Virginia.

And coincidentally, (I like to say that a lot), today is my 33rd-week surviving GBM. How nice is that!

I started to write my own simple Obituary. I have arranged to have my body donated to Life Legacy Foundation; they have a program with the University of Miami, which accepts brains for study. They can study my brain and the rest of my body for up to six months, after which it will be cremated and sent back to Delynn in an Urn. Delynn's mother, who died of GBM, had donated her body to science. It's a good thing. My soul will be in Heaven. My body will continue to help science. Then I will be consigned to the flames just as it should be.

Until then, I've got six weeks or less to finish the Chronicles. Electronic reorders on!

Delynn notes: It was interesting that David wrote the above experience and thoughts as on the same day I sent an email to David's sisters. March 13, 2016.

Hello, I did not include your mom in this email, as I do not want to upset her. I will leave that to your discretion.

I know we spoke on Friday about some of this, but after our night last night, David did fall and also had soiled himself without realizing it had happened. He was unable to help transfer himself to and from the potty seat. He had been able to do this just a few days ago.

And after speaking with a few people from Hospice about David's symptoms and decline, including the RN, I remembered we had this site that talks about the difference between this type of cancer and other cancers or general dying when it comes to the decline and timeline.

Many of the 3 to 6-week symptoms are happening to him. Some are on the list of 2 to 3 weeks, but his mind, as we know, is very brilliant may take much longer to decline. He has had no interest in going anywhere, even out of bed, to the porch or sitting up. Yes, partly because of the dizziness, but partly he is ambivalent. I guess it is part of the symptoms.

Here is there link

http://www.brainhospice.com/SymptomTimeline.html

I hope this helps as we all prepare for what we don't want to prepare for.

Always in prayer!!

Delynn

18

The Timekeeper

Until We Meet Again

On a delayed train from Manchester to London in 1990, JK Rowling wrote her first idea for the Harry Potter series on a napkin. She typed her first book, *Harry Potter and the Philosopher's Stone* (later published in America as the Sorcerer's Stone) on a typewriter, often choosing to write in many of the Edinburgh Café's.

Sitting at Nick's Restaurant just after sunrise, coffee cup in hand, I sometimes felt like Rowling. My writing task surely was much simpler on a modern laptop than Rowling's old manual typewriter. Even though I learned to type on the old IBM Selectric in the early 1980s, I can't imagine how much longer this book would have taken typing on the ancient machines. As many times as I have iterated, deleted, moved paragraphs, filed, spell corrected, and backspaced, I found great respect for the writers of the late 19th and 20th centuries who wrote and got published. They must have been infinitely more organized, and their minds trained entirely differently to write the way they did. I can only imagine they must have thrown a lot of crumpled paper into the trash bin before they typed, *"The End!"*

I ate at Nick's Restaurant every morning the last six months, almost always ordered breakfast, usually the "Pooch," for $3.50. Two poached eggs, one slice of grilled tomato, and applesauce instead of potatoes. It became a meal I looked forward to every day. The breakfast named after its owner, Pooch, opened up the little hole-in-the-wall at 7:00 a.m., the '60s and 70s music playing lightly overhead and Fox News jabbering over their refrigerator just made writing a little easier.

I almost always had my laptop and leather journal open, and in-between bites of food, intently writing or typing.

Eventually, curiosity got the better of him. He asked, "What do you write about?"

Before I said anything, I asked Valerie, my favorite breakfast waitress, to refill my coffee. Not as simple as it sounds, but Valerie made it simple. She picked up the hot water pot in one hand and the coffee pot in the other and poured them together into my cup without hesitation. I tore open five half n half creamers and made my diluted coffee white. Wimpy coffee. But it was my ritual.

I talked to Pooch about my cancer, near-death experiences, and my race to finish and publish the book. He was sitting on a bar stool with his one-year-old granddaughter on his lap, feeding her scrambled eggs. He had Dead Saint stories to tell, just like nearly everyone I talk to.

To this day, I still believe that Francisco, Nick's elder dishwater and busboy, was an angel in disguise who smiled asked me every day how my book was going.

NDEs and Cancer in the Payment Industry

I wonder how the payment world will respond to my death. With disinterest? Or will they be curious? Over the years, I have watched a few payment industry friends die from cancer. Sam Caine, who wrote *The Silver Linings of Cancer*, died from Throat cancer in 2013, a few months after my cancer discovery. I emailed Sam the first chapter of my book about NDE's a month before he died. I hope he had a chance to read it. Another payment industry giant, who negotiated a major contract I had, died in July 2009 at 62, after a six-month battle with GBM.

Unfortunately, another payment industry CEO, Colin Reed, recently discovered he has GBM. He just finished 33 standard radiation treatments and has begun Chemo. Delynn has been in constant contact with his wife to walk her through what we already know he will experience. *He died three months after David.

Other industry friends have confided in me about their own Dead Saint experiences. One friend shared he'd collapsed on the restaurant floor from a deadly reaction to seafood and viewed his dying body from above. He hired me as a payment consultant for his company after my non-compete expired in 2014. As we began to know each other better, he found out about my book and then told me his NDE story. He, too, is a saint. I am sure he will cringe when he sees this.

Fast Transact's success created a "good name" for me in what sometimes can be a less than honorable business, a business I had always tried to make proper. As a result, I hope to reach thousands of my payment industry friends who have wondered about Heaven and life after death.

Perhaps, God looks down from Heaven and wonders if I will decide to live, or if I will decide it's my time to die. Sometimes I think I have chosen, and at other times I wonder.

When I bring up the possibility to others that I may be approaching my "appointed time," I get push back. God can heal anything! Don't think that way! You are pointing the bony finger of death at yourself!

Sighhh. I know inside it is a balance between always keeping the will to live versus knowing when "my time" is approaching. We all die. It is not a failure to pass. I know God has a plan, and I must continue to do my part for as long as possible.

Have I released my burden? Have I let go of my remorse? My guilt? Paul Solomon used to describe letting go to be as simple as a child who climbed a little too high in a tree and is hanging onto a branch afraid to let go and fall the few feet to the ground. His father reaches up to him and says, "Let go, son, I will catch you!" It's the easiest thing to do, but it seems at the same time the hardest thing to do.

Is there life after death? I can say with absolute conviction. Yes! I can say this because I have had my own experience of the Afterlife, of Jesus Christ and eleven deceased friends and family who have visited me in dreams. Or when Jesus' electric presence blasted me in my living room in 2011 or had me kneeling on an NYC sidewalk in 1981. I did not imagine that. I didn't expect it or evoke it with my imagination. It just happened. A spiritual existence which changed my life.

All the Afterlife anecdotes are reassuring. Doubt is always the twin brother of Faith. Faith grows when there is less doubt. When you have a direct experience of God, then Faith leaps exponentially to KNOWING. It's that simple.

Delynn thinks I'll never rest. She says that I complain that there is always too much to do and so little time to do it and too many things I still need to learn. I lament that I don't spend enough time with my children and wife. I have run the race for nearly three years and most of my time focused on completing the Chronicles. I feel I need to reach out to those who have lost loved ones and share my experiences. I would like to finish the telescope I started grinding in 1975, and I would like to see my daughter, Angela, graduate High School in June 2016.

These are my desires.

Delynn has walked beside me throughout this journey and has been instrumental in writing, editing, scanning, and smiling. She props me up when I was ready to fall; she pushed me forward when I wanted to give up. She thinks I am still too hard on myself, but that most likely will never change.

I've thrown everything but the Afterlife kitchen sink at you. I hope my work and my stories have helped guide you through the vast uncharted territories revealing vistas and realms previously unknown or misunderstood. Maybe you feel more confident about what happens when you die. Does Heaven feel more real?

Do you feel you are a part of God's Plan? That you are here to make a difference? You are still on a Mission from God. Watch and listen to your dreams. Watch why things happen when they happen.

Keep a journal and keep this book handy. Pass it along to your friends.

Do not be afraid.

I feel the *Chronicles* has built a bridge to the Afterlife you can walk across without fear. With an absolute conviction that the Living One, Jesus Christ, the Creator, the Divine One is real and approachable. There is nothing that can keep you from the love of God.

It is my prayer all faiths come to recognize the wisdom of the Dead Saints and seek out their Holy conversations with God. Perhaps, in our lifetime, science will prove life after death exists. Maybe then religious leaders will take another look at their Holy Books with new eyes, not to cast them aside, but to help clarify the writings of their own ancient teachings.

Perhaps a unifying Gospel will be written by a prophet who walks and talks with God in our generation; a visionary who helps us recognize what is real and what is false; what is true and what is an illusion; a prophet who shows us, Heaven, inside and Heaven outside.

A prophet who personifies love and kindness. A prophet who will recognize Christ when He comes again.

The rest of this story is a Heavenly masterpiece, painted by thousands of Apostles, disciples, Saints, and Dead Saints throughout time to make complicated something truly very simple. Immortality is your inheritance. Eternal life is Christ's gift. Heaven is just a smile away. If you think you've done something so horrible that God would reject you, I want you to trust God. The Creator is not so small. He wants you to grow up and learn that love IS the only WAY. He will forgive all things, no matter what. No matter what, my friend. Even after death. That's all you need to remember. That's all you need to know.

How much time do I have left? God will give me exactly enough time to finish what I came here to do. When God is finished with me, then I will be allowed to leave.

Until then, I will continue to write through my scribe and lovely wife, Delynn. Her trials as a caregiver for me have been exhaustive. GBM is not easy, and she hasn't gotten to the hard part yet. Whenever I need just a moment of compassion, she says, "I'm sorry. I'm sorry you're feeling this way." Just taking a moment to recognize my pain is all I need.

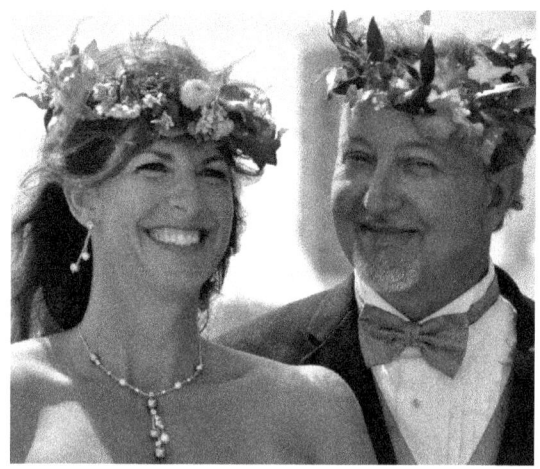

Delynn is one of the most amazing souls I have ever known. She is my "Commanding Heart." I think she is the girl I dreamed about when I was 16, who prostrated beside me before Jesus Christ committing to finishing the work he asked us to do. What a love story! She has done that and much more.

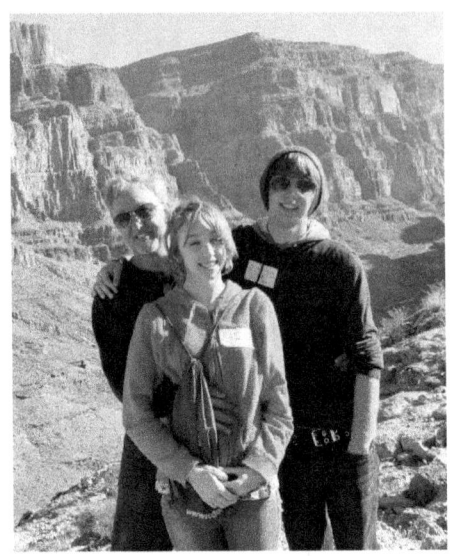

What Do I Say to my Children?

And lastly, what do I say to my children? I will say how much I love you and how dear you are to me. Do you remember camping and my truck piled high with bicycles? Do you remember singing songs from the Shrek CD at the top of our lungs in Kauai? And floating around the Grand Wailea water park? All these memories and so many more. I wish I could be here for you

Angela and Ben when you graduate college or land a great career. I wish I could be there at your wedding, and see the birth of your first child. To you both, I pray you find a job and a career that is something you truly love, and not work you are required to do to make a living. If you can, start your own business, and be in charge of your own lives, just as your mother and I did.

Ben, I remember when the nurses placed you under the warming lights in the hospital crib minutes after you were born. I watched your body relax, like you were under a hot tropical sun. I followed you everywhere throughout the hospital so I would not lose sight of you.

When we went home, so you would not cry all night, I placed you on my chest and belly to calm you, so we both could sleep. I spent the next year playing with you all the time because I was busy writing my book at home.

I remember the night when you were two years old, you excitedly jumped up and down on the bed and pointed at the ceiling. "Mommy, Daddy, birdies!! Birdies!! Birdie for Mommy, Birdie for Daddy, Birdie for Benamin." (not misspelled) I believe angels visited us that very night.

You were wise beyond your years, confounding your baby sitters and school teachers. Ben, you still are wise, you are still sweet, and you are loving. Don't worry about failure or success. Just be yourself. Tell no white lies and keep your promises. Prepare for the future as I have told you, for the changes are coming sooner and will be more dramatic than you think.

Angela, I remember delivering you at birth with the assistance of Dr. Hurd. Your mother had three previous miscarriages, and she had to have her cervix tied, just to keep you in the womb to be born. You were determined to be here. I remember telling you night time stories almost every night to cull you to sleep. Stories of the bouncing ball that bounced higher and higher until it escaped Earth's gravity, bouncing ever higher until it reached Jupiter, and then falling again to be capture by us in our house. Or the Ant Story and its journey throughout the house captivated by the wonders of all the "big things" it saw in its travel around window sills, doorways, furniture, and toys.

Angela, you are so good, thoughtful and loving. You do some silly things from time to time, but we all have done that. Especially, Daddy. You have a sharp, clever, creative mind. Your music should become a part of your life no matter what.

You'll be able to do whatever you set your heart on doing. Keep on singing and playing your beautiful music forever!

I'm sorry I wasn't always there for you when I built our Company. We needed to pay bills, and the stress of building it, took over my life, my heart, and my focus away from you. It was not my intention to go after the "diamond," but that's what I did. Not on purpose, but by accident. Don't let future careers or business do that to you. Pay a LOT of attention to your kids and your spouse. Family and love are all that really matters. The rest is just stuff.

Above all, I pray you both find your own experience of Jesus Christ. He is very approachable, a regular Joe kind of guy. During times of trouble, just talk to him as you would any friend. And then watch what happens. Make it a science experiment. Repeat the experiment. It's the cry of the heart demanding a response that will come in His TIME.

Nothing I can say write will change your beliefs until you experience His presence. Until then, if you can, have Faith. The Planetary Headmaster and His angels are watching over you.

The Chronicles are my legacy, and they are dedicated to you. There is nothing for either of you to ever fear, because I too, will be watching from above, and should those in charge allow, I will visit you in your dreams.

I love you both so much.

It pains me more than you know that I leave you so young. Losing Dad will hurt for a while. Time and tears heal, but death always leaves scars. There is a reason for everything, and later in life, you may come to know why God allowed this experience to happen, how it impacts you, and maybe you'll understand why God took me away.

Always remember you are extraordinary. Be of good cheer! We will meet again. Until then, be good. Love one another. Dad.

The communication from the Dead Saints has always been, "There is a preferred path." Even Christ had to choose to give up His free will and recognize the Preferred Path His Father desired.

It is a choice to apply our free will, but aligning our choices, and there are many, to the will of the Father and following the "still small voice" an easier task once I have committed to don the Mind of Christ. Then all the Christ within who is one with the Being of Light and Jesus Christ without, all the Saints, archangels, angels, Rice Paper teachers, will withdrawn swords will without hesitation, protect and guide you. A stairway of angels leading from Earth to the Holy City in Heaven. Jacob's ladder.

To all the Saints, my family, and friends. May His peace be with you until we see each other again in Paradise.

19

The Timepiece

Dorothy's Hour Glass

~Delynn, who likes to be prepared early for everything, called Hospice today. They need a doctor's order to start the process. The first step is for a Hospice staff member to come by and make an assessment of my condition. It's a common dilemma with GBM caregivers. When to call Hospice? Those afraid of death wait too long. Those anxious about treatment call too early. I think it's a bit too early, but my physical condition has been deteriorating weekly and is one of the signs to "get ready" because weekly decline becomes daily decline. The call seemed easy, but her tears showed otherwise. For me, I feel like an observer. I don't feel like I am going to die soon. I feel no fear. I just keep on typing, even though I know Dorothy's hourglass is running out of sand. February 29, 2016. ~**Chronicle 992**

Delynn notes: As I was completing the last chapters to send off to a publisher, I was looking through documents, notes, letters, and journals to make sure I could remember as many details as possible what was transpiring during David's final days.

In 2016 and 2017, I made attempts to complete this work but was thwarted by many obstacles. I wasn't ready. I was still processing my grief, which honestly never truly leaves. Yet, this year, I feel I have been led to finish the books. It is encouraging to know when you are being guided when the doors open up to you, and you determine you must keep going.

In 2016 I had attempted to work on both of David's books. Of course, this one being the hardest to complete. Even as I send for publishing, so many things could have stayed in or been taken out. There were so many miracles, blessings, and even hard to discuss moments that could have gone into this book. It is heartfelt for sure.

David's third book, the *Armageddon Stones*. I opened up in 2016 as well, thinking I could review it and maybe find a co-author. I found a manuscript that needed editing and writing to the point I had no hope of either editing or finding someone who could piece together the book's vision. Then in May of this year, 2020, I was going through a bunch of files and found a near-completed version he had worked on up until just days before he passed away. It was nearly complete!

Due to its complexity, cost, and cognition, the 3rd book, *ARMAGEDDON STONES,* is being published simultaneously, in its unedited version for those who want to learn and build upon its knowledge.

David had also transcribed his journals and continued to make his journal entries into a Word document.

I'd discovered his last edit was on April 15th, just three days before passing; he also had set his word doc journal to dates out to April 24th, 2016. He had a calendar set out to Chronicle 1101, June 18, 2016- Angela's graduation from Cox. April 2nd was his last journal entry:

~ My shriveled legs look like a WWII Holocaust victim. I hadn't really notice. I am peeing constantly every 15 minutes, so the Hospice nurses use a sticky condom fitting device over my private parts instead of a catheter. It's amazing how much urine my body discharges. Delynn has to empty a full urine bag 3x a day. The liquid is coming out of my leg muscles.

The Hospice nurse told me about another GBM patient who is going through the same thing with his legs, but he has had GBM only 8 months. Like me, he has some upper body strength, but we cannot stand or walk. I get another of Delynn's hot showers in the kitchen tomorrow.

Rumors, I am on my deathbed, are running amok! I am still taking radio interviews! Mind as sharp as a tack! Lot's to do! April 2, 2016. ~Chronicle 1025

David's "real" pain began about two weeks before 3:10 a.m. April 18th, 2016. He had not been able to walk unassisted since March 11th, the hospice bed was being used, and the makeshift shower had been implemented. He was unable to tell when he was urinating. We were having to change him regularly. He was no longer able to turn over by himself. It was getting more difficult. He thought it was time to have a catheter so he wouldn't hurt himself trying to get up.

A hospice nurse came to insert the cath, and it appeared to be painful for David. At the time, I had no idea how they worked, so I had not considered there may be a problem. Ben and I watched while the nurse waited to see the urine go into the bag. During this time, David was saying the pain was excruciating; he was crying.

The nurse finally realized she had not inserted it far enough and had inflated the ball. It was inserted again, and a third time, finally, we had urine in the bag. From that time on, David's pain almost non-stop.

It was the same week David's published book came in. We had ordered 300 books to be shipped to us; the rest was kept at the printing company's distribution center. Finding and organizing the space, organizing the book signing, and the many interviews scheduled. Our publicist Dotty and her team were working non-stop.

He was set to live stream on Saturday with the local IANDS group, and the next day would be the live streaming to the Fellowship of the Inner Light. By the 9th, we were already told there was not an infection. He was in pain.

He'd just completed a live stream talk with the VBIANDS: the Virginia Beach chapter of the International Association of Near-Death Studies. The meeting was held at the A.R.E. about a mile from where we lived, but David was propped up in his hospice bed to complete the live stream interview about his first book. We had planned for a book signing a few hours after the live stream.

As soon as he was done with the live streaming, he was in tears, and we didn't know what to do. I called hospice, who had already been at the house the same day. They said it would be hours before they could come back. Karie Alton, who had been at the A.R.E., had come to the house for the book signing.

She had the time incorrect, so she arrived early. Just in time to help calm David and hold his hand while I asked hospice for instructions to take out the cath, which seemed to be causing so much pain. The hospice nurse walked me through the steps. It seemed to release some of the problems, and David was able to relax.

There was a good attendance for the book signing. David did, however, become very tired, and it was time for sleep.

He needed to rest because we were doing another live streaming with the Fellowship of the Inner Light the next day. It was the Sunday before he passed.

We believed he had an infection, which hospice scheduled a test to be performed on Monday. They said he did not have any type of infection, urine, bladder, or otherwise. Something was still amiss.

By Wednesday, he could not tolerate the pain, so I called for an ambulance to take David to the emergency room. He needed some relief.

His mother joined me at the hospital. They did numerous tests, and he had, in fact, had a severe bladder infection. They helped provide some relief for him.

He was sent home with a different pain medicine regimen; instead of morphine, the emergency room doctor prescribed him Dilaudid. Though sometimes morphine is better for pain, some people respond to Dilaudid. She said we should not mix the two.

Once we returned home, he was able to sleep better.

Besides our hospice nurses, Ben, my sister-in-law Sue, David's mom, and I helped with his care. He no longer had feelings in the lower half of his body. He wasn't able to tell when he needed help. My brother was to return on the 19th to take my sister-in-law home. She had been with me for three weeks and needed to return home. My long-time friend, Jacky, had arrived on the 16th to help.

I remember Jacky walking into the room, David smiling and being so happy to see her and saying, "You look like Jesus." She was my true blessing, and always my sister in Christ.

Early about 2:00 am on the 16th of April, David asked me to help him end his life. He never thought he would find himself saying this. But here it was. I was stunned and wasn't sure what to say. I wanted to relieve him of his pain. I wanted him healed. I wanted so badly to help him. Yet, I knew this wasn't what he wanted. I said, "David, I will agree to help you if you first tell both your children that you want to do this." It took everything I had to make that statement.

Mentioning his kids made him come out of his mind and pain and thought that no, he would press through.

I knew his time was coming to an end. I was thankful to have Jacky there. She was a caregiver and knew what was happening.

The next morning my son called asking about David. I told him I didn't think he would be here long, and if he wanted to come up from Georgia, it would be nice. James arrived at the house that night. He and David had a special connection, for which I am forever grateful.

The next evening at about 2:00 am on the 17th of April, David again called me over to his bed, but this time told me: "It's time and let's do it today" I was again stunned, yet could see it was time. I sent an email to a few of his closest friends that said:

> Hello, Beloveds,
>
> David's health has declined significantly over the last few weeks and more so in the last week. He has said he would like to go home today. Early on the 16th he was struggling with great pain and asked for help in leaving. A difficult request to hear and was able to help relieve some of the pain with the help of hospice. His breathing and ability to keep his lungs clear is becoming more difficult. At about 2 am he said "It's time and let's do it today" Not in a chipper way but more that he is just ready.
>
> I am not sure what time or how or even if but desire to ask for your assistance for him to transition. I know the norm is to ask for assistance and prayer in staying yet he says he is ready. I want to honor his wishes to the extent I am to do and all I can do is pray.
>
> Much love, Delynn

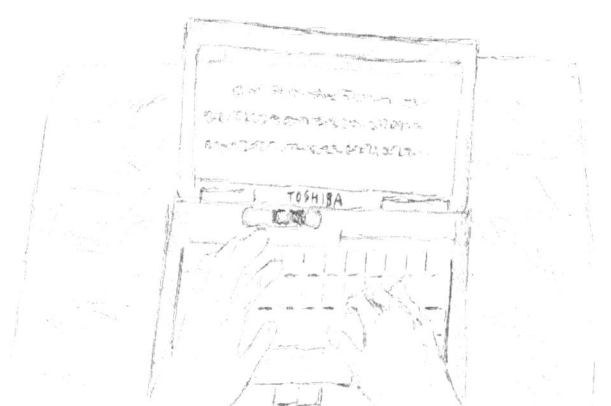

Days earlier, he had been reorganizing and completing the *Armageddon Stones*. He didn't want to stop typing. He was typing to the point his wrists were getting sores because he was unable to lift them. I tried to find something that would work, then decided to cut the top band area of thick winter socks. It worked perfectly. He was signing books and editing both *Training Wires* and *Armageddon Stone* as of Friday the 15th. He had received two interviews requests, one was with a subsidiary of Guidepost, which made us excited, yet I replied that we would have to wait until Monday to see how he was feeling.

By late afternoon on the 17th, David was in constant pain, moaning, and laboring. All I could do was hold his hand and pray. I honestly felt like he was transitioning, with laboring pains, birthing to the other side.

There were quite a few people in the home throughout the day. David's mom, Ben, James, myself, Jackie, and Sue had been there continually throughout the day. Angela had gone back to her aunt's home. We were at a loss as to how to comfort him. Hospice had been in and decided he needed to switch back to the Morphine instead of the Dilaudid. We were not sure what was best. Jacky had recognized his body was what they called "mottling."

I knew David said he was going today, yet I was not sure. I held it in my heart, wondering. Would he have that experience he spoke of that he and God could change this course around.

Word had begun to spread and I began to get more emails, for both David and me. I read what I could to David and responded to those I'd emailed at 3:10 am with an updated email:

> Thank you all. In short because too much gratitude and response to share at the moment. He had asked to have Hallelujah played continually in concert with the seven terrace. So we are doing that. He is mostly out with a lot of mottling and hospice said it could be today or next few. Family is gathering around. I'm praying its today for him because it's a beautiful day here in Virginia and the sparrows have been singing all day. The large azaleas are in bloom with the colors of the terrace in them. We are surrounded by all the beauty this world can offer and thankful for that.
>
> His daughter also came and spent time with him and also sang hallelujah to him and her own song she wrote for him. He was alert enough to talk to her briefly.
>
> There has been wonderful help all around these last few weeks through so many people, and more coming in, though it still is hard to see him hurting even when you have all the help around. We are giving him diladid 4mg every 3 hrs with adavan (sp) and a little more in between when needed.
>
> Also read your, Stephen's, eulogy to him. He wasn't able to respond but know he heard every word. And felt good.
>
> Going to lie next to him for a while and do the seven terrace.
>
> Love Delynn

The hospice nurse had come again to assist. We wanted to relieve his continual paid but didn't want to give him too much. She was there about midnight; she was with us for a few hours then left, telling us to provide him with a dose of the pain relievers every hour. She left, and everyone went to bed; it was just past 2:00 am. Everyone decided to get some rest.

David's mom had stayed. She and I were going to sleep in the bed next to him. I had the Murphy bed set up next to his hospice bed to sleep next to him. I would hold his hand every night or lay my hand on his chest.

I sent out a few emails, including this email sent at 2:54 a.m.:

David continues to labor. His laboring, at one point, reminded me of labor in birthing. I was thinking he is birthing himself to the other side. And then giving him assistance with the help of hospice and now morphine/adavant every hour. Thank you for talking with David and your love. Received the beautiful letters from your boys and was able to share them with David. I need to get an hour of sleep before next meds. Xoxox! Delynn Solomon

Our church still had people coming daily to help. I needed to respond to Francis Spore's email (Francis created our log for our books).

Mon, April 18, 2016 1:42 a.m.

Hello, Delynn and David, I hope things are going OK over there! Esp after Susan's announcement today! God's will be done...As you know, I'm supposed to bring you food at midday, and I'm fully prepared to do that, but if there's any change of plans, or special requests, please let me know

ASAP if you can! What I'm planning to bring is homemade chicken meatball soup with raviolis in it, too, and chopped celery and carrots as well. Also some fresh cooked asparagus and an apple cobbler-type (whole grain) dessert.

Mixed baby spring mix salad, as well. (I assume you would have favorite dressings there? Hard to second guess that). If any of this is a problem, let me know -- again if you can. I was planning to get an autographed copy of David's book today. Just FYI. I had held off knowing I would be coming over today. My prayers and energy are with you. Strongly...Love, Francis

At 3:03 am I responded: Mon, Apr 18, 2016 3:03 AM to FSporer

Francis, yes feel free to come by and looking forward to the meal, only because you made it sound so wonderful, though David will not be able to eat any of it. Myself and our family would.

I am so sorry to say that unless David has a rally he is not able to sign any books. We do have a book here for you. Very tired. Look forward guy seeing you in the morning. We have our own salad dressing. Delynn Solomon

Less than 5 minutes later, we realized the oxygen machine was still running even though the hospice nurse had taken it off him the hour before, saying he was getting enough oxygen. I got up and shut it off. Getting comfortable again, ready to close my eyes,

I rolled over to put my hand on David's chest as I did every night. I felt him and did not feel him moving. I held my own breath, wondering if his breathing rate had slowed down, but there wasn't any movement. I turned to his mother and said, "David's not breathing." She quickly jumped up and went to the other side of his bed. We both realized he was not here anymore. I blurted out, "Congratulations, David." David's mom said, "You snuck out on us." It was 3:10 a.m. April 18, 2020.

My head was reeling. He labored so hard all day, so many of us standing with him, wondering if he would go at a particular moment or would he be here a few days longer. He had visitors earlier in the day. And now, after everyone had gone to bed 30 minutes prior, with the only sound of the oxygen machine running and once that was turned off and all quiet, he left.

It's like he waited for everyone to calm down for him to go. I went upstairs and got Ben first, then woke the rest of the house. I called the hospice nurse to see what we needed to do next; they connected us with the funeral home. Our friend, Larry Jennings, was a funeral director. He made the arrangements to prepare David's body to be donated to the university. The mortuary men came to take his body.

I was still in shock, not realizing I still had decisions to make. My parents had died in a hospice care unit, and I had no idea about the procedure. They came and asked what clothes we would like to put him in. I hadn't even thought about that!! Well, I knew instantly he would want to be in his new silk robe; it was his replacement after having worn Paul Solomon's silk robe for many years. I quickly went upstairs to get the robe. I kept the sash.

They didn't want us in the room while preparing his body and taking him to the funeral home. I'm not sure if I even cried that night. I'm not sure if I was even breathing. I do know I was in a state of shock.

Everything seemed either in slow motion or a blank movement. They took the hospice bed that morning. The Murphy bed was folded up, and the living room looked like a living room again. It was surreal. We really were not expecting him to die, not right then. It didn't seem possible. Yes, all the signs were there. Yes, I was glad he was not feeling any pain. He was gone, and I was lost.

Francis knocked on the door. He had lunch in his hand and, as always, his big smile.

Appendix B
The Garden Scroll

My heart is a garden called Eden. My garden is fertile and productive. The seeds that fall into my garden need only a little encouragement to flower. Like Eden of old, my garden is a blessing or a curse. A fertile garden untended becomes a jungle and there is not garden more fertile than the garden of my heart and my mind.

If weeds and thistles were planted, it would be weeds and thistle that grow. Neither weeds nor thistle will disturb the flowers of my heart that bring joy to my life. The Ancient One said, "As a man thinks in his heart, so is he." What I have planted in the garden is what I am or is what I think I am, and all that I ever may experience of life is what I plant in the garden of my heart.

I will avoid the seeds of hurt and pain that would blemish the beauty of my garden. Neither seeds of doubt, nor thorns of hurt, nor thistle of self-pity will be my experience of life.

I am a gardener. My heart is a garden tended by my mind. Whether heart or mind, my garden is the place where I have planted words, thoughts, beliefs and ideas. These seeds have been cultivated long and have produced the fruit that is the way I see and experience the world.

I am a gardener, thinker, and creator. My feelings come from my garden. My words and my thoughts plant seeds that determine wither weeds or flowers will thrive there. My actions and reactions, my emotions, and my habits will plough and cultivate, water and feed the plants that grow in the garden of my heart.

Like all men and women, I talk to myself. My mind is active each waking moment and my mind is filled with words, thoughts and opinions. This day I declare these thoughts and opinions shall be my own. What I plant in my garden is my own choice and I will carefully cultivate the highest and best fruits of wisdom.

My words and my thoughts, my opinions and beliefs are both produce from my garden and they are the seeds and the compost that feed my garden again and again. The plants that grow there, whether good or bad, become stronger, more deeply rooted; more pervasive every day. Today, I choose only good seed to plant in the fertile ground of my heart.

The untended garden is filled with beliefs, habits, and interpretations. A facial expression or an unkind word can feed hurt in the garden of thistles and weeds. I will be alright with myself. I will choose not to plant weeds of judgment sown by unkindness. When one is unkind and disapproving of me, I will take responsibility for my own self-worth. I will give myself praise when I need it most.

Life is about what is and I accept that. I do not wish for what should be. It is not always fair but never more than I can endure. Whatever shall come, I will say, "I can handle it," and handle it I will, for my garden shall thrive and I will be happy.

I have not always been aware of thoughts and influences that designed the garden of my heart and mind. I was not always aware that confidence, self-esteem and the experience of being loved planted beautiful flowers instead of weeds.

Now I know the truth. I am the master gardener of my life. I now take charge of what I tell myself. I am responsible for the thoughts that determine what I believe. The way I feel every day is a direct result of what I tell myself and what I have told myself time and time again.

If, at first, it seems difficult to say loving and wonderful things about myself, my loved ones, and my life, it is because this one little flower of self-worth I plant today would have been choked by the thousands, yea millions of weeds I planted and fed with past thoughts, but this flower will survive – I have decided it!

Today I plant a new garden. It is a garden of joy and new life. The produce of my garden is health, prosperity, love and kindness. My garden feeds me with abundant and nourishing relationships. Laughter and contentment will fruit in the garden of my heart. Each new thought of love, repeated over and over, will replace old habits and thought patterns sown in fear. Where once there were weeds and thistles of fear, resentment, and anger, choking my garden, there are now flowers of love, forgiveness, and peace, transforming the garden of my heart and mind into Heavenly place.

How shall I succeed? The difference in those who fail and those who succeed lies in changing destructive thought habits into supportive thought habits.

When I was a child, I spoke as a child, I understood as a child, I thought as a child. Now I am grown and I put away childish things. When I was a child, I was influenced by others. I became enslaved to their beliefs and habits. Where I was a slave to impulses, I also became a slave to habits. When I felt worthless, it was because I was criticized. My low self-esteem was starved for praise. I depended on others and what they said about me to feel alright.

Now I am my own. I no longer depend upon approval from others. My habits are mine and I give myself approval. I will not starve for love. I will feed myself with love, with self-worth and self-esteem. It is not longer for others to establish my worth. It is my responsibility and I am able to respond. I am not a slave to old habits.

My habits are my own and they are a choice. I am a deciding being with my own free will and I have decided this day to plant seeds of self-worth and self-esteem.

I once surrendered my free will to self-defeating habits. The years of cumulated guilt and years of bad habits may have already marked a path through my garden which would have threatened my future. A victim is ruled by appetite, passion, prejudice, greed, love, fear, environment, and habits—and the worst of these tyrants is habit. I will neither be a slave or victim. I will be master of my fate. Old habits pass away, behold all things become new. Thus I know the law which precedes all others; I will form good habits and obey their commands.

I believe what I tell myself, as I always have. I give myself praise and support. I encourage myself and my future. This is an effortless path. If it seems difficult, I will make it effortless by my commitment. Until I am committed, there is hesitancy.

I will drop the shackles of doubt and commit myself in this very moment to begin a new life, for I know that boldness has genius and power to make it so.

My commitment is made; my beginning is now.

Through reading this scroll, my new life has begun. This scroll will plant new seeds of joyous, positive, loving and healthy thoughts I want to plant in my garden.

It is one of nature's laws that only a habit can replace another habit. For these words to perform their chosen task, I must discipline myself with the first of my new habits, which is as follows:

Each day I will feed my mind, heart, my garden, even as I feed my physical body, for forty days and nights. I will read the words in silence when I arise to assure that the "seed thoughts" of my day, will establish my mood and expectations, will be nourishing, healing thoughts that will lift me to God, the Source of My Being.

I will read the scroll in silence at mid-day before taking my meal to feed the strong roots of new habits growing in my garden. And before I retire at days' end, I will read the scroll ALOUD so that I will fall asleep with the "seed thoughts" I choose for my beautiful garden. On the next day, I will repeat this procedure, and I will continue in like manner for forty days and forty nights.

And what will I accomplish with this habit? Herein lies the hidden secret of all man's accomplishment: my every action directly results from the way I think.

And from where will come my help?

My help comes from God, my Source, the source of my mind, my body, and my spirit. I will make my Source, my Inner Teacher, a personal friend, and turn my thoughts to that Source at least three times a day. As I read the words daily, they become a part of my conscious mind. But more importantly, they will also seep into the rest of my mind, that mysterious part which never sleeps, which creates my dreams, and often makes me act in ways I do not comprehend. My lower and lesser mind will become obedient to my Higher Mind rather than to my old appetites and old habits.

As the words of this scroll are consumed and digested by the depths of my mind, I will begin to awake each morning with a vitality I have never known before. My vigor will increase, my enthusiasm will rise, my desire to meet the world will overcome every fear I once knew at sunrise, and I will be happier than I ever believed possible.

I will find myself responding to all situations that confront me as I commanded myself in this scroll to respond. These actions and responses will become effortless and natural, for any act with practice becomes easy.

Thus a new and good habit is born in both thought and action. Every act is a direct result of the way I think. My original thoughts and actions become a pleasure to perform through repetition. And if they are a pleasure to perform, it is my nature to perform them often. When I perform them often, they will become a habit and begin to serve me. This is my will.

I make a solemn oath to myself that nothing will retard my new life's growth. I will lose not a day from reading this scroll, for no day can be retrieved, nor can I substitute another for it. I must not, I will not break this habit of daily reading for forty days, for in truth, and the few moments spent each day on this new habit are but a small price to pay for the happiness and prosperity that will be mine.

Today new wisdom is planted in the garden of my heart. I commit myself this day. I am succeeding.

And for this, I give.

OBITUARY: DAVID BEN SOLOMON
APRIL 18, 2016

David Ben Solomon passed away at home surrounded by his loving family in the early morning hours on Sunday, April 18, 2016. Born in Novato, California on January 23, 1959 to Ronald Bruce Early and Annalee Joan Gregory, David grew up in Virginia Beach, Virginia and graduated from Princess Anne High School in 1977. David served in the United States Airforce as a B-52 Gunner before becoming a full-time apprentice to Paul Solomon for 15 years from 1979-1994. David documented Paul's life during world tours to Egypt, Israel, Europe, Australia and Japan. During this period of teaching and apprenticeship, David studied under many teachers gaining his knowledge and wisdom of the art of Bonsai, and Tai Chi, all of which he loved. In 1992 and 2010, Solomon assisted Egyptologist John Anthony West and geologist Dr. Robert M. Schock in re-dating the Sphinx, as well as other Egyptian and Turkish monuments, proving them many thousands of years older than previously thought. David's earlier extensive comet impact research supported the re-dating of these ancient sites. In 1994, he appeared in a supportive role on the national telecast NBC special Ancient Prophecies II, where he discussed the life and prophecies of Paul Solomon, founder of the Fellowship of the Inner Light, where David was also an ordained pastor.

After Paul Solomon's death in March 1994, David moved to Washington State and retired; from spiritual studies to build a family and business. There, he founded Fast Transact, Inc. Over the next 15 years; the company became one of the largest online payment processing companies in the Pacific Northwest. In January 2010, with the sale of the company, David returned to his spiritual roots and created Akio Botanical Japanese Gardens, bringing his love of bonsai to his surroundings and his life. In July 2011, as the Japanese gardens transformed his property, David began intensive research into the near-death experience, a project he would subsequently call The Dead Saints Chronicles.

His research was 95 percent complete when he was diagnosed with Glioblastoma Multiforme IV (GBM), a rare, aggressive brain cancer that kills 50 percent of its victims within 15 to 18 months. Thirty-four months after the diagnosis, David fulfilled his dream of bringing his 1st book, The Zen Journey Through the Christian Afterlife, to print on April 6th. His book is the first in a trilogy with the second and third books: Training Wires of the Soul and The Armageddon Stones, which will be published later this year. Along with his mother and father, left to cherish his memory are his wife, Delynn Carol Solomon; his children, Benjamin Solomon, and Angela Solomon; stepson, James Thayer; his stepdaughter, Leah (Jason) Hughes; and his step-grandchildren, Aiden, Liam and Mila; his sisters: Michelle (David), Terri (John) Marko; and many nieces and nephews, all of whom he loved. He was preceded in death by his stepfather, Ray W. Gregory.